Muscle Building

Elevating Your Fitness and Transforming Your Body

(Essential Guide to Building the Body Muscles for Great Performance)

Larry Bethea

Published By **Cathy Nedrow**

Larry Bethea

All Rights Reserved

Muscle Building: Elevating Your Fitness and Transforming Your Body (Essential Guide to Building the Body Muscles for Great Performance)

ISBN 978-1-7776902-3-6

No part of this guidebook shall be reproduced in any form without permission in writing from the publisher except in the case of brief quotations embodied in critical articles or reviews.

Legal & Disclaimer

The information contained in this book is not designed to replace or take the place of any form of medicine or professional medical advice. The information in this book has been provided for educational & entertainment purposes only.

The information contained in this book has been compiled from sources deemed reliable, and it is accurate to the best of the Author's knowledge; however, the Author cannot guarantee its accuracy and validity and cannot be held liable for any errors or omissions. Changes are periodically made to this book. You must consult your doctor or get professional medical advice before using any of the suggested remedies, techniques, or information in this book.

Upon using the information contained in this book, you agree to hold harmless the Author from and against any damages, costs, and expenses, including any legal fees potentially resulting from the application of any of the information provided by this guide. This disclaimer applies to any damages or injury caused by the use and application, whether directly or indirectly, of any advice or information presented, whether for breach of contract, tort, negligence, personal injury, criminal intent, or under any other cause of action.

You agree to accept all risks of using the information presented inside this book. You need to consult a professional medical practitioner in order to ensure you are both able and healthy enough to participate in this program.

Table Of Contents

Chapter 1: Understanding the Science of Muscle Growth 1

Chapter 2: Building a Muscle Growth Training Program 11

Chapter 3: Sculpting a Muscular Back 27

Chapter 4: Creating Strong Legs 39

Chapter 5: Maximizing Muscle Growth with Advanced Training Techniques 52

Chapter 6: Tracking Your Progress and Making Adjustments 65

Chapter 7: Maintaining Motivation and Discipline 73

Chapter 8: The Science Behind Muscle Building 86

Chapter 9: The Role of Protein Synthesis 97

Chapter 10: Optimizing Recovery for Faster Muscle Growth 105

Chapter 11: Avoiding Common Mistakes 122

Chapter 12: Muscle Mass Building 135

Chapter 13: Anatomy and Physiology ... 140

Chapter 14: Designing Your Training Program 152

Chapter 15: Progressive Overload and Training Intensity 163

Chapter 16: The Perfect Repetition and Technique 174

Chapter 17: Training Frequency and Recovery 182

Chapter 1: Understanding the Science of Muscle Growth

For a few years, people have been enthralled with the search for a toned frame and accelerated power. The method of gaining greater muscle organizations and energy is known as muscle increase. It is a complex phenomenon associated with the delicate interaction of severa physiological processes. This chapter delves into the technological expertise of muscle increase, studying the crucial thoughts that manual this existence-converting phenomenon.

Anatomy of the Muscle

Sarcomeres, the primary constructing blocks of muscle fibers, are contractile devices that make-up muscular tissues. Actin and myosin are the 2 primary protein filament kinds located in sarcomeres. Actin and myosin filaments skip past each different in reaction to a signal from the hectic device, producing a contractile strain that permits muscle groups to shorten and settlement.

Mechanisms of Growth in Muscle

1. Hypertrophy: The increase of man or woman muscle fibers leading to a median growth in muscle tissues is referred to as hypertrophy. There are critical strategies with the resource of which this happens:

Myofibillar Hypertrophy: term "myofibrillar hypertrophy" refers back to the growth of sarcomeres, or contractile devices, in each muscle fiber.

Sarcoplasmic hypertrophy: This circumstance is characterised through way of manner of an boom in the quantity of sarcoplasm, the fluid that surrounds every muscle fiber's contractile components.

2. Hyperplasia: The term "hyperplasia" refers to the boom of muscle fibers inside a muscle. The primary mechanism for that is the activation of satellite television for pc tv for pc cells, which is probably muscle stem cells

in a latent state with the potential to proliferate and differentiate into new muscle fibers.

Elements Affecting the Growth of Muscle

1.   Training Stimulus: The crucial stimulus for muscle increase is resistance education, which includes making use of an outside strain to muscle corporations. Training quantity, frequency, and intensity all have a large impact on the development of muscular hypertrophy.

2.   Hormonal Response: Growth hormone and testosterone are essential hormones that contribute to muscular growth. These hormones assist muscle corporations adapt and mend with the useful aid of selling the synthesis of muscle proteins.

three. Nutrition: Getting the electricity and building blocks desired for muscle growth calls for a healthy healthy dietweight-reduction plan. For the increase and restore of muscle mass, protein, carbs, and wholesome fats are all vital vitamins.

four. Recovery: After exercise, muscle corporations need to get keep of sufficient time to relaxation and regenerate. Growth hormone and unique hormones concerned in muscle increase are released during sleep.

The Function of Progressive Overload

Establishing present day overload is essential for constructing muscle. It is the idea that to typically check muscle groups and promote increase, the training stimulus need to be step by step accelerated over time. You can accomplish this with the resource of way of running out greater frequently, lifting heavier weights, or doing greater repetitions.

Maximizing the Growth of Muscle

The following procedures have to be considered to optimize muscle increase:

1. Emphasis on Compound moves: Give particular hobby to compound movements

like squats, deadlifts, bench presses, and rows that art work for numerous muscular agencies proper away.

2. Maintain Correct Form: To reduce accidents and boom muscular activation, proper shape and method are vital.

three. Include Training Variations: To provide your muscle groups with various stimuli, strive the usage of education techniques like drop gadgets, supersets, and big devices.

four. Eat Enough Protein: To promote muscle growth and restore, intention for 0.8–1 grams of protein in step with pound of body weight every day.

five. Make Sleep a Priority: To assist your frame heal and regenerate, try to get 7-8 hours of accurate sleep every night time.

6. Handle Stress: Learn actual coping mechanisms for coping with stress, as extended-term strain can impair muscular increase.

Recall that developing muscle is a sluggish manner that calls for regular paintings, strength of mind, and a wholesome food regimen.

Accept the Process and Get Amazing Outcomes

By comprehending the ideas of muscle growth, setting into workout green training techniques, and maintaining a health-aware manner of living, you may set out on a remodeling path to attaining your physical objectives. Accept the issues, recognize the accomplishments, and be conscious the terrific metamorphosis that occurs whilst you expand your power and body.

The Role of Nutrition in Muscle Building

When you begin your adventure toward a properly-defined frame, you may find out that food plan is truly as crucial as workout. Your muscle companies require the right vitamins to develop and repair themselves, similar to an vehicle wishes fuel to operate. We'll dive into the dietary ideas in this financial damage to help you gas your fitness quest and attain your whole muscle-constructing capability.

The Protein Mysteries: The Components Required for Muscle Growth

The building block of muscular development is protein. It is the crucial detail that your muscular tissues require to regenerate and mend following resistance schooling. Microscopic tears are produced at the same time as hobby breaks skeletal muscle fibers. The amino acids included in protein assist to repair those tears, which results in large and more potent muscles.

The Function of Carbohydrates: The Energy Source for Muscle Growth

In the arena of fitness, carbohydrates are from time to time misinterpreted, although they may be important for developing muscle. They supply your muscles the strength they require for strenuous workout as well as to heal and expand. Although structural increase requires protein, carbs offer your muscle groups the nourishment they need to perform at their excellent.

The Importance of Good Fats: The Silent Heroes of Muscle Growth

Good fat, frequently maligned for being linked to weight benefit, are important for building muscle and keeping favored health. They encourage the synthesis of hormones, in particular testosterone, that is essential for the boom of muscle. Furthermore, appropriate fats aid exceptional cell function and the absorption of vitamins.

Micronutrients: The Unsung Heroes of Muscle Growth and Their Significance

Although they may be regularly neglected, vitamins and minerals are examples of micronutrients which might be important for each stylish fitness and muscular constructing. As co-factors in severa biochemical techniques, vitamins and minerals ensure your body works at its pleasant to assist the increase of muscle.

The Timing of Meals: Maximizing Nutrient Utilization

The time you eat has a massive have an impact on on how an awful lot muscle you advantage. Before an workout, eating protein and carbohydrates offers your muscular tissues the power they require to function at their top. Consuming protein and carbohydrates after an exercising quickens the way of muscle increase and repair.

Supplements Function: Strengthening Your Nutritional Basis

The majority of your nutritional needs have to be met through way of manner of a balanced eating regimen, notwithstanding the truth that supplements can provide a similarly enhance. If you've got hassle getting enough protein from weight loss program alone, protein nutritional nutritional supplements like whey protein can also help you satisfy your each day protein goals. It has been confirmed that the frame's natural deliver of creatine will boom muscle increase and feature.

Crafting a Nutrition Plan for Muscle Growth

Your healthy dietweight-reduction plan should be custom designed to satisfy your particular wishes and goals. When calculating your intake of protein, carbohydrates, and fat, consider your frame weight, quantity of hobby, and training program. To create a customized nutritional plan that will help you gain your muscle-constructing objectives, talk with a licensed dietitian or nutritionist.

Chapter 2: Building a Muscle Growth Training Program

A well-organized training software program is your road map to success as you obtain down to builds a muscular body. We'll discover the basics of designing a a achievement education plan on this chapter, providing you with the tools to create a time table that fits your goals, diploma of health, and way of life.

Understanding Your Training Goals

Setting education goals is critical earlier than deciding on physical video video games and set/rep schemes. Is your purpose to growth widespread strength, hypertrophy of the muscle companies, or each? Setting precise objectives let you track your improvement and direct your training software.

Choosing Complex Exercises: The Cornerstone of Muscle Growth

The foundation of any training software geared inside the course of developing muscle is compound wearing sports or actions that artwork for plenty muscle businesses proper away. They beautify wellknown power and provide the most powerful stimulus for muscular growth. Examples encompass rows, bench presses, deadlifts, and squats.

Incorporating Isolation Exercises: Refining Muscle Definition

Exercises that isolate specific muscle corporations can enhance fashionable appearance and help outline muscle mass more exactly. But in preference to taking the location of complex workouts, they need to beautify them. Lateral will increase, tricep extensions, and bicep curls are a few examples.

Determining Set and Rep Schemes: The Muscle Growth Language

The quantity of units and repetitions you whole for each exercise is decided with the resource of set and rep schemes. It is typically cautioned to do pretty a few eight–12 repetitions for three-5 units to growth muscle groups. This range permits sufficient recuperation time in among sets and offers enough stimulus for muscular increase.

Gradual Overload: The Secret to Continuous Growth

The mystery to ongoing muscle increase is progressive overload, or growing workout quantity or intensity frequently through the years. To encourage continued increase, you need to task your body greater even as it will become aware about your present exercising stimulus.

Training Frequency: Finding the Correct Balance

The range of instances each week that you educate a specific muscle organisation is known as training frequency. Even while training extra often can result in quicker improvement, it's crucial to provide yourself enough time to rest in amongst intervals. It's enough for beginners for beginners to exercising consultation each muscle company to 3 times consistent with week. You can up the frequency of your exercise to a few to 4 times per week as you broaden.

Rest and Recuperation: The Unheralded Heroes of Building Muscle

For muscular tissues to develop, rest and rehabilitation are clearly as vital as actual education. Your muscle groups grow huge and more potent due to self-restore at some stage in sleep. For the satisfactory feasible recuperation, a wholesome diet regime, enough sleep, and lively recuperation techniques like foam rolling and stretching are critical.

Customizing Your Exercise Program to Fit Your Lifestyle

Your exercise ordinary want to art work along aspect it slow desk and way of life. If time is of the essence, consciousness on compound sports and provide precedence to overall performance. For more muscle definition, keep in mind doing greater isolation bodily video games in case you are extra bendy.

Monitoring Your Development: Assessing Your Achievement

It's vital to tune your development to hold motivation and adjust your schooling routine. Record the quantity of weight you elevate, the variety of repetitions you complete, and the general quantity of power you construct. Utilize this records to evaluate your development and make any corrections.

Establishing a Durable Training Schedule

Sustainable muscular boom is crucial for long-term success. Select a workout ordinary that you live up for and may stick with over time. Try a preference of things to determine what works top notch for you.

Recall that developing a muscular frame is a journey rather than a race. Accept the method, stay steadfast in your objectives, and take delight within the first-rate metamorphosis that takes place as your frame is shaped right proper right into a monument to your determination and the technology of muscle building.

Overcoming Common Training Plateaus

You may also experience plateaus as you flow into in advance with your muscle-constructing endeavors; those are instances at the same time as your development stops or slows down significantly. Although they'll be disturbing and demoralizing, the ones plateaus are a ordinary component of the education way. This bankruptcy will speak frequent motives for training plateaus and offer viable solutions that will help you damage thru them and boost up your muscle boom.

Recognizing Training Plateau Symptoms

Recognizing the lifestyles of a education plateau is step one within the route of conquering it. The following are normal signs that you is probably at a standstill:

No Strength Gains: You have not located a discernible boom in strength after lifting the same weights for a few weeks or months.

Muscle Definition Stalls: Despite normal workout, your muscle tissues no longer look like turning into more defined.

Reduced Motivation: You be conscious that your normal is boring or unchallenging, and you are dropping the selection to train.

Knowing What Leads to Training Plateaus

Training plateaus can be due to numerous things:

Absence of Progressive Overload: Your frame adjusts and ceases responding to the stimuli in case you do no longer gradually increase the amount or depth of your exercising exercises.

Poor Nutrition: Too little protein or too few energy would possibly probably prevent muscle corporations from growing and getting better.

Overtraining: Training an excessive amount of without enough restoration time can placed on you out, lessen your overall performance, and lift your danger of harm.

Stress: Prolonged strain can prevent the synthesis of hormones and the recuperation of muscular tissues, that would avoid your potential to benefit muscle.

Lifestyle Factors: A lack of sleep, horrible nice of sleep, and wonderful manner of life alternatives might also in all likelihood restriction the boom of muscle.

Techniques for Breaking Through Training Plateaus

After you've got determined the probably motives for your stagnation, it's miles essential to vicinity the ones techniques into exercising:

Boost Progressive Overload: Increasing the burden you enhance, the quantity of reps you do, or the style of devices you end want to all be finished regularly.

Optimize Nutrition: Make positive you've got become enough strength and protein in your eating regimen to assist with muscle growth and restore.

Make Rest and Recovery Your Top Priority: Give your muscle tissues enough time to get better and expand in among durations.

Reduce Stress: To lower pressure ranges, try strain-good buy techniques like yoga, meditation, or time spent in nature.

Change Up Your Training Routine: To push your muscle groups in novel ways, attempt introducing new workout workouts, adjustments, or schooling techniques.

Seek Professional Advice: For individualized recommendation, reflect onconsideration on speaking with a licensed non-public instructor or dietitian.

Preventive Steps to Prevent Training Plateaus

Include the following sporting events to your education regimen to avoid hitting a plateau within the future:

Track Your Progress Often: Keep a watch on your ordinary overall performance, frame composition, and electricity profits to grow to be privy to plateaus early on.

Periodize Your Training: To maximize muscle boom and recuperation, combo at some stage in times of stepped forward and reduced schooling depth.

Emphasize Sleep: To sell latest health and muscular restore, purpose for 7-eight hours of correct sleep every night time.

Maintain a Healthy Lifestyle: To enhance elegant properly-being, manipulate pressure stages, devour a balanced weight-reduction plan, and get common workout.

Recall that plateaus are not a barricade, but as an alternative a temporary hassle. You can get past those obstacles and preserve on with your quest for a toned body with the resource of comprehending the reasons, placing beneficial techniques into exercising, and which includes preventative measures. Accept the problems, preserve your integrity, and take pleasure within the remarkable exchange you've got finished with commitment and staying power.

Building a Strong Chest

As the dominant characteristic of your better body, your chest is a instance of energy and athleticism. A properly-described chest is a favored bodily reason for masses people as it radiates self warranty and strength. This bankruptcy will take you on a adventure to bring together a nicely-described, muscular chest. We'll discover the mind and sports as a way to turn your pectoral muscle agencies right right into a assertion of your willpower.

The Anatomy of Your Chest

Your pectoralis primary and pectoralis minor are the principle muscle groups for your chest which may be concerned in flexion, adduction, and inner rotation of the chest. They are vital to many movements, along side pulling, pushing, and throwing.

The Science of Building Chest Muscle

Your chest muscle agencies enlarge through a way called hypertrophy, or the increase of muscle cells, much like any other muscle. Resistance training starts this device by way of putting pressure for your muscular tissues, which ends up in their breakdown. Your muscle groups heal themselves at some degree within the restoration phase, growing bigger and stronger as a stop end result.

Crucial Exercises to Develop a Strong Chest

Incorporate those physical games into your software program program to get a powerful chest:

1.   Barbell Bench Press: The entire chest, triceps, and anterior deltoids are labored in some unspecified time in the future of this compound exercising.

2. Dumbbell Bench Press: wider chest muscular fibers are activated via this model, which gives you a much wider kind of motion.

three. Incline Dumbbell Press: This workout promotes a more first-rate higher chest through highlighting the higher segment of the chest.

four. Decline Dumbbell Press: This version strengthens the entire chest with the resource of focusing on the decrease chest.

5. Dumbbell Flyes: This isolation workout enables to break up muscle companies via using focusing on the chest location.

6. Push-ups: This body weight exercising can be adjusted to in shape various levels of fitness and is a superb way to growth chest energy.

7. Cable Crossovers: This remoted workout lets in to define the contour of the chest by means of using highlighting the inner a part of the chest.

Instructional Guidelines for Ideal Chest Growth

To optimize chest growth, adhere to the following hints:

1. Aim for eight-12 repetitions constant with set: For maximum appropriate muscle growth, cause for 8–12 repetitions constant with set. This range offers really enough stimulus to purpose tiredness.

2. Complete 3 to 5 gadgets of every exercising: This quantity allows enough muscle boom and activation.

three. Rest for 30-ninety seconds amongst units: Take a 30-to-90-2nd damage in among gadgets to provide your muscle tissue a threat to heal before the following exercise.

4. Include revolutionary overload: To hold your muscle tissues challenged, step by step growth the weight you carry or the quantity of repetitions you do over time.

5. Keep appropriate form: To reduce damage and increase muscle activation, right shape is crucial.

Nutrition and Recuperation for the Development of the Chest

Growth of the chest muscle depends severely on nutrients and recovery:

1. Consume sufficient protein: Eat enough protein because it includes the constructing blocks preferred for muscular boom and repair. One gram of protein in step with pound of frame weight want to be your each day motive.

2. Ensure ok carbohydrate intake: Make first rate you have grow to be sufficient carbohydrates because of the fact they offer you with the energy you need to perform active exercising. Try to devour 45–sixty five% of your each day power as carbs.

three. Prioritize sleep: Make sleep a topic as it's throughout sleep that muscle tissue increase and mend. Make an try to attain seven or eight hours of real sleep every night time.

4. Include lively rehabilitation: Blood go together with the waft and muscle repair may be extra effective through easy wearing activities like yoga or taking walks.

Embrace the Chest Development Journey

A sturdy chest can only be completed with determination, workout, and the proper form. Accept the revel in, enjoy the paintings, and notice how your chest miraculously adjustments to become a example of your tenacity and remedy.

Chapter 3: Sculpting a Muscular Back

A strong and athletic body is characterized through a properly-advanced once more, which is an indication of electricity, manipulate, and backbone. This monetary damage will communicate the technology of muscle boom, the structure of the lower again, and the exercise exercises and techniques as a way to show your once more right right into a sculpture of flawlessly normal muscle.

Anatomy of the Back: The Basis for Strength

Your lower back is fabricated from an complicated net of muscle mass, every of which has a distinct feature in posture, stability, and movement. The following are the principle lower back muscle companies:

1. Lastissimus dorsi(lays): The biggest muscles in the lower back, the latissimus dorsi, or lats, are accountable for pulling motions and assist create a first-rate, V-commonplace lower back.

2. Trapezius(traps): The trapezius, or traps, bypass from the neck to the mid-once more. They beneficial resource shoulder motions and help create a extensive, robust higher again.

3. Rhomboids: These muscle mass, which is probably located inside the location between the shoulder blades, useful resource in pulling the shoulders once more and assist a nicely-described, muscular higher decrease back.

4. Erector spinae: Located along the backbone, those muscle corporations useful resource and stabilize extraordinary moves of the backbone.

The Science of Back Muscle Growth: Exposing the Mechanisms

Like all muscular boom, the method of hypertrophy is accompanied via the growth of the lower once more muscle mass. Resistance training places pressure on your decrease back muscle companies, that could lead to small rips. Your muscle organizations get larger and more potent because of self-restore and rebuilding within the route of the recuperation diploma.

Key Exercises to Develop Sculpture inside the Back

Incorporate the ones sports into your software program to growth a muscular returned:

1. Pull-ups: This complex exercising works the rhomboids, lats, and traps, which enhances lower returned increase everyday.

2. Bent-over rows: This version concentrates at the center lower back at the identical time as working the lats, traps, and rhomboids.

three. Seated cable rows: This form of isolation exercise allows to separate muscular tissues and desires the lats.

4. Face pulls: This exercise improves better once more definition via focusing on the rhomboids and rear deltoids.

5. Deadlifts: The lats, traps, erector spinae, and hamstrings are all worked in the course of this compound exercise.

6. Barbell rows: This version emphasizes the top lower back on the identical time as operating the lats, traps, and rhomboids.

7. T-bar rows: This exercise works the lats and traps at the identical time as supplying a impartial grip that lessens wrist stress.

Training Guidelines for Optimal Back Development

Take word of these pointers to optimize again improvement:

1. Aim for eight–12 repetitions constant with set. This range gives definitely enough stimulus to cause tiredness.

2. Complete three-five sets of each workout: This amount permits enough muscle increase and activation.

3. Rest 30-to-ninety 2d between units. To gift your muscle groups a hazard to heal in advance than the subsequent exercise.

four. Include revolutionary overload: To preserve your muscular tissues challenged, regularly boom the burden you bring or the range of repetitions you do over time.

five. Keep nicely shape: To limit harm and boom muscle activation, proper form is important.

6. Concentrate on the mind-muscle connection: During your exercise, be aware about the muscle tissue you are the use of and contract them deliberately to increase muscular activation.

Nutrition and Recovery for Back Development

Growth of the once more muscle is based upon significantly on vitamins and healing:

1.   Eat enough protein: because it consists of the building blocks favored for muscular increase and restore. One gram of protein in step with pound of frame weight have to be your every day motive.

2.   Ensure adequate carbohydrate consumption: Make certain you are becoming sufficient carbohydrates due to the fact they provide you with the strength you want to perform full of existence exercising. Try to eat forty five–sixty 5% of your each day power as carbs.

three. Prioritize sleep: Make sleep a priority as it's in a few unspecified time in the destiny of sleep that muscles increase and mend. Make an effort to reap seven or eight hours of real sleep each night time time time.

four.   Include lively rehabilitation: Blood waft and muscle repair may be greater appropriate by means of using easy physical video games like yoga or strolling.

Embrace the Journey Back Development

To growth a muscular again, one should be devoted, continual, and use the proper shape. Accept the experience, take pleasure within the manner, and word your once more magically change into an great example of power and strength.

Developing Powerful Arms

Your fingers are the physical instance of your power, strength, and agility, and they will be vital to each day with the resource of day duties and athletic achievement. This chapter will address the technological information of muscle growth, the anatomy of the arms, and the exercise exercises and strategies on the manner to turn your fingers right into a lovely instance of your dedication to tough paintings and resolution.

Anatomy of the Arms: Understanding the Framework

Your palms encompass 3 vital muscle groups:

1. Biceps brachii: The biceps, which are decided on the the the front of the top arm,

are in charge of forearm supination and elbow flexion.

2.	Triceps brachii: The triceps, that are positioned on the rear of the pinnacle arm, are concerned in elbow extension further to the general duration and energy of the arm.

3.	Forearms: Made up of loads of muscle groups, the forearms are in rate of gripping, wrist flexion and extension, and finger moves.

The Science of Arm Muscle Growing: Exposing the Mechanisms

Like all muscle increase, arm muscle boom proceeds via the hypertrophy manner. Your arm muscle groups are careworn all through resistance exercise, which leads to minute rips. Your muscle agencies get larger and stronger due to self-repair and rebuilding in the end of the healing degree.

Essential Exercises for Powerful Arms

Incorporate those wearing sports activities into your software to develop robust palms:

1.   Barbell Bicep Curls: This is a complex workout that develops the biceps average by focused on them.

2.   Hammer Curls: This version specializes in the brachialis, a deeper muscle within the biceps that permits define and increase the biceps.

three. Inclined dumbbell curls: This exercising develops the biceps' top region and enables to outline the bicep peak.

4.   Triceps Pushdowns: This shape of isolation exercise develops the triceps normally with the useful useful resource of specializing in them.

five.   Extensions of the Overhead Triceps: This version complements the length of the triceps head, which allows outline and sculpt the triceps.

6.   Close-Grip Bench Presses: This compound exercising strengthens and develops the palms preferred with the

resource of the use of focusing on the triceps and anterior deltoids.

7. Wrist Curls: This remoted exercise improves grip energy and forearm definition by way of manner of manner of focusing at the forearm flexors.

eight. Reverse Wrist Curls: This model strengthens and defines the forearms thru focusing at the extensors.

Training Guidelines for Optimal Arm Development

Take be privy to these tips to optimize arm improvement:

1. Aim for 8–12 repetitions in step with set. This range gives honestly sufficient stimulus to reason tiredness.

2. Perform three-four sets of each exercise: this amount will help your muscle tissues to boom and spark off properly.

3. Rest three-four gadgets in step with workout: Take a 30- to 60-2nd harm in among

devices to give your muscle organizations a hazard to heal earlier than the following one.

four. Include current overload: To preserve your muscle groups challenged, regularly increase the weight you increase or the sort of repetitions you do over time.

5. Keep specific shape: To reduce harm and boom muscle activation, right form is essential.

6. Concentrate on the thoughts-muscle connection: During your exercise, take note of the muscle organizations you are the usage of and settlement them intentionally to boom muscular activation.

Nutrition and Recovery for Development of Arms

Recovery and nutrients are vital for constructing arm muscle:

1. Eat enough protein: as it consists of the building blocks desired for muscular boom and repair. One gram of protein normal with

pound of body weight must be your every day purpose.

2. Ensure good enough carbohydrate intake: Make effective you are getting enough carbohydrates because of the reality they come up with the electricity you need to perform lively exercising. Try to devour 45–sixty 5% of your each day electricity as carbs.

three. Prioritize sleep: Make sleep a trouble as it's inside the direction of sleep that muscle mass increase and mend. Make an attempt to gain seven or eight hours of suitable sleep every night time.

Chapter 4: Creating Strong Legs

The cornerstone of your present day energy, persistence, and athleticism is your legs, the powerhouse of your frame. They are critical for lots one-of-a-kind types of hobby, consisting of jumping and sprinting, lifting heavy items, and doing every day chores. This bankruptcy will speak the generation of muscle growth, the anatomy of the legs, and the exercising sports and strategies on the way to turn your legs right right into a effective and ambitious image.

Anatomy of the Leg: Understanding the Framework

There are numerous crucial muscle businesses for your legs:

1. Quadriceps(quads): The quadriceps, or "quads," are the muscle tissues in front of the thigh which can be concerned in knee extension further to the general energy and duration of the legs.

2. Hamstrings: The hamstrings, which are discovered in the rear of the thigh, are concerned in hip extension and knee flexion, which complements leg power, energy, and athleticism.

three. Calves: The calves, which may be determined inside the rear of the decrease leg, are in price of plantar flexion, which lets in you to propel your self off the floor whether you run, soar, or stroll.

4. Adductors: The muscular tissues that pull the legs collectively throughout adduction are located at the inner thighs.

five. Abductors: The muscle tissue at the outside of the thighs are in charge of abduction, that is the movement of the legs apart.

The Science of Leg Muscle Growth: Exposing the Mechanisms

Like all muscle increase, the way of hypertrophy is accompanied by means of the increase of leg muscle. Your leg muscle corporations are forced within the route of resistance workout, which leads to small rips. Your muscles get large and stronger because of self-restore and rebuilding inside the route of the healing diploma.

Crucial Exercises to Develop Strong Legs

Incorporate those wearing sports into your software program to growth effective legs:

1. Barbell Squats: This compound workout strengthens and tones the quads, hamstrings, glutes, and center further to the legs.

2. Leg Press: This variation enhances barbell squats via providing a slightly extraordinary attitude for activating the quadriceps.

3. Deadlifts: This compound workout improves large leg energy, energy, and posterior chain improvement through using focusing at the hamstrings, glutes, and lower decrease lower back.

four. Leg Extensions: This remoted exercising promotes quadriceps period and definition thru manner of emphasizing the quadriceps.

5. Curls with the hamstrings: This is an isolation exercising that strengthens and could increase the scale of the hamstrings.

6. Calf Raises: Exercises for the calves, which includes calf will increase, decorate calf energy and definition.

7. Lunges: This exercise improves leg energy, power, and balance via focusing at the quads, hamstrings, glutes, and middle.

8. Step-ups: This exercise strengthens and tones the quadriceps, hamstrings, glutes, and calves.

Training Guidelines for Optimal Leg Development

To optimize leg improvement, adhere to the subsequent suggestions:

1. Try to stick to 6–12 repetitions consistent with set; this variety permits for enough recuperation time similarly to supplying enough stimulus for muscular boom.

2. Perform three-4 gadgets of each exercising; this quantity will help your muscle organizations to make bigger and set off well.

3. Rest for 30-60 seconds among units: Take a 30- to 60-2d spoil in amongst units to offer your muscle businesses a risk to heal before the following one.

four. Incorporate modern overload: To preserve your muscle tissues challenged, grade by grade boom the burden you raise or the range of repetitions you do over the years.

five. Keep pinnacle shape: To reduce damage and growth muscle activation, proper shape is vital.

6. Concentrate at the mind-muscle connection: During your exercise, be aware of

the muscles you are using and agreement them intentionally to boom muscular activation.

Nutrition and Recovery for the Development of Legs

Growth of leg muscle groups is based upon extensively on diet and recovery:

1. Consume enough protein: Eat sufficient protein as it includes the building blocks wanted for muscular growth and repair. One gram of protein in step with pound of frame weight must be your each day intention.

2. Ensure proper sufficient carbohydrate intake: Make first rate you are becoming sufficient carbohydrates due to the fact they arrive up with the electricity you need to carry out energetic workout. Try to consume forty five–sixty 5% of your daily energy as carbs.

3. Prioritize sleep: Make sleep a topic because it's at some point of sleep that

muscle businesses grow and mend. Make an try and gain seven or 8 hours of excellent sleep each night.

4. Incorporate active rehabilitation: Blood go with the flow and muscle restore may be advanced with the aid of clean wearing activities like yoga or taking walks.

Embrace the Journey of Leg Development

Proper technique, strength of mind, and consistency are critical for developing powerful legs. Accept the task, respect the paintings, and notice how your legs will miraculously alternate as you shape them into a base of energy, energy, and athleticism.

Enhancing Core Strength and Stability

Your body's powerhouse, your middle, offers the framework for all-spherical health, electricity, and stability. It includes the muscles to your back, hips, and stomach that assist your spine, guard your inner organs, and provide you the strength to do some of sports activities. This bankruptcy will cowl the significance of middle stability and energy, in addition to practical sports activities and strategies to decorate your center feature.

The Importance of Stability and Core Strength

A robust and regular center is vital for:

1. Injury Prevention: Better spinal resource from a strong middle lowers the hazard of once more ache and harm from every day sports sports and sports.

2. Enhanced Athletic Performance: A robust middle enhances energy transfer, balance, and coordination, which benefits lots of sports sports sports and sports.

three. Better Posture: Maintaining precise posture eases the pressure at the back, shoulders, and neck. This is made feasible with the aid of a strong center.

4. Daily responsibilities: Having a strong center makes it much much less difficult to carry out every day responsibilities

collectively with bending, twisting, and sporting gadgets.

Essential Exercises for Stability and Core Strength

1. Plank: This isometric exercising strengthens and stabilizes the complete center.

2. Side Plank: This model improves center balance and definition through focusing on the obliques, or the muscular tissues on the edges of the stomach.

three. Bird Dog: This exercising works the muscular tissues in the lower once more, shoulders, and hips at the same time as improving middle stability and coordination.

4. Crunches: This exercising strengthens and defines the belly muscle groups through focusing on the rectus abdominis, moreover referred to as the "six-%" muscle.

5. Russian Twists: This workout improves rotational balance and definition by using using the obliques and middle muscle groups.

6. Bicycle Crunches: This version complements hip flexion and center stability at the same time as focused on the rectus abdominis and obliques.

7. Dead Bugs: This workout improves spinal stabilization, middle balance, and coordination.

8. Superman: This workout improves middle balance thru way of strengthening the posterior chain muscle businesses, which encompass the back and glutes.

Training Guidelines for Core Strength and Stability

To optimize your center energy and balance, adhere to the subsequent tips:

1. Include middle sporting activities to your software. To efficaciously offer a lift to

and stabilize your center, purpose for 2-3 middle workout routines normal with week.

2. Keep suitable form: To restriction harm and increase muscle activation, right form is critical.

3. Pay hobby to the mind-muscle connection: During each exercise, consciously agreement your middle muscle groups.

4. Progress frequently: Make incremental improvement by means of the usage of beginning with fewer weights or fewer repetitions and little by little growing the depth over the years.

5. Pay interest in your frame. Steer clear of overtraining and take days off while critical to permit your frame heal.

Nutrition and Recovery for Stability and Core Strength

Core muscle boom and regeneration are supported with the aid of the use of appropriate healthy dietweight-reduction plan and recovery:

1. Eat enough protein: because it includes the building blocks desired for muscular increase and restore. Your each day cause need to be zero.Eight–1 grams of protein in step with pound of body weight.

2. Ensure precise sufficient carbohydrate consumption: Make superb you are getting enough carbohydrates due to the fact they help with muscle recuperation and come up with energy for exercising. Try to consume forty five–sixty five% of your every day calories as carbs.

3. Make sleep a topic. Sleep is crucial for the increase and restore of muscle groups. Make an try to acquire seven or eight hours of authentic sleep each night.

four. Include lively restoration: Simple sporting activities that increase blood go together with the flow, which incorporates yoga or taking walks, can assist muscles get higher.

5. Drink enough water: Sufficient hydration is essential for every favored health and muscle performance. Throughout the day, make it a issue to stay hydrated.

Embrace the Journey of Stability and Core Strength

Improving balance and center power is an ongoing technique that needs commitment and regularity. Welcome the journey, get satisfaction from the art work, and watch as your center undergoes an wonderful metamorphosis at the same time as you installation a sturdy base for your normal fitness, power, and power. Recall that a body with a sturdy middle may additionally moreover accomplish first-rate feats of power and performance.

Chapter 5: Maximizing Muscle Growth with Advanced Training Techniques

You can experience a plateau to your muscle-constructing adventure, wherein your earnings prevent or slow down. This is wherein more modern schooling techniques are beneficial because of the truth they provide a unique stimulus to push your muscle groups and encourage endured development. This bankruptcy will cowl severa advanced education strategies that will help you get the most from your schooling and growth the amount of muscle you could gain.

1. Drop Sets: Overcoming Weakness for Ongoing Development

Drop devices entail regularly lowering the burden you improve on the equal time as maintaining the rep rely number consistent. By using this method, you may push the set past your everyday component of failure, which keeps your muscle agencies developing even while you're exhausted.

Example: Use 50 pounds to perform eight reps of bicep curls. As quickly as you begin to feel tired, lessen the weight to 45 pounds and do three or four greater reps. Once again, carry out this exercising with the load decreased to 40 pounds for two to three repetitions.

2. Supersets: Maximizing Muscle Fiber Activation

Two bodily games are finished another time-to-returned in a superset with little to no ruin in amongst. By that specialize in numerous muscle companies or muscle fibers, this technique maximizes the activation of muscle fibers and fosters widespread growth.

Example: Do eight barbell squat reps, and then eight leg press repetitions right after. After a 30-second smash, repeat the cycle three or 4 times.

3. Giant Sets: Pushing Your Limits for Maximum Growth

Giant units encompass chaining collectively many workout exercises concentrated on the equal muscle region with minimal recovery between them. By straining your muscle tissues to their breaking thing, this method promotes speedy muscle growth.

Example: do 10 barbell curl repeats, ten hammer curl repetitions right away, and ten awareness curl reps. After a 60-2nd harm, repeat the cycle three or 4 times.

four. Taking Advantage of Post-Tetanic Potentiation in Rest-Pause Training

A set of an exercise, a brief wreck, and then every extraordinary set till failure include rest-pause education. Post-tetanic potentiation, a physiological phenomenon with a purpose to increase muscular contractility following a quick relaxation, is used on this technique.

Example: bench press 8 instances. After a fifteen-2d destroy, repeat the preceding set of 8 reps. Go via this manner once more, trying to finish three units in preferred.

5. Progressive Overload: The Basis for Muscle Growth

Muscle increase is primarily based totally on current overload, this is the current increase in education load over time. Your muscles are constantly located to the test, which makes them more potent and extra adaptable.

Example: Increase the weight you improve or the quantity of repetitions you do in dumbbell presses as you benefit more potent. This developing workload will hold promoting muscular boom.

Incorporating Advanced Techniques Strategically

Considering your expertise diploma, schooling targets, and capability to get properly, you need to cautiously maintain in thoughts incorporating superior education techniques into your routine. One or techniques at a time to start with, and as you end up extra used, regularly up the intensity.

Recall that to prevent harm and maximize effects, using superior strategies requires nicely shape and relaxation.

Accept the Challenge and Enjoy the Benefits

Cutting-issue schooling strategies can provide your efforts to acquire muscle a massive enhance, allowing you to overcome plateaus and make excellent development. Accept the task, skip past your consolation region, and enjoy the blessings of a stronger, extra toned frame.

Enhancing Muscle Recovery and Injury Prevention

Making muscle restoration and damage prevention your pinnacle priorities even as starting your muscle-building adventure is important. These factors are critical for optimizing your outcomes, reducing setbacks, and ensuring that you can hold up your fine schooling. This financial disaster will cope with strategies to hurry up muscle repair and defend your body from harm that could prevent your growth.

The Significance of Muscle Recovery

The gadget by means of using which your muscle tissues regenerate and mend after an workout consultation is referred to as muscle restoration. Your muscle fibers maintain small tears while you perform resistance bodily video video games. Although these tears are essential for the development of muscle, furthermore they want enough time to heal.

Strategies for Effective Muscle Recovery

1.   Make sleep a subject. Try to get 7-eight hours of suitable sleep each night time time. While you sleep, your frame releases chemical compounds that promote muscle growth and restore.

2.   Eat the Right Foods: Make top notch you are getting enough protein and carbs to help rebuild your muscle tissue and offer you with strength on your next exercise.

3.   Include Active restoration: To increase blood flow and facilitate muscular healing, soak up moderate exercising at the facet of yoga, swimming, or taking walks.

4.   Apply Foam Rolling and Stretching: These strategies can help in decreasing pain, developing flexibility, and releasing muscle anxiety.

five. Think About Post-Workout Supplements: Protein powder and creatine are examples of nutritional nutritional supplements that could beneficial useful resource in muscle building and recovery.

Techniques for Preventing Injuries

1.   Warm-up Before Every Workout: Every exercising need to start with an splendid warmness-as plenty as get your muscle groups organized for motion and reduce your chance of damage.

2.   Preserve Proper Form: Maintaining proper shape in some unspecified time in the future of workout is essential to averting joint

problems, strained muscle groups, and famous physical strain.

3. Listen to Your Body: Pay Attention to Any Pain or Discomfiture That Your Body May Feel. If a few aspect feels incorrect, surrender the workout and, if desired, get help from a professional.

4. Prevent Overtraining: Take sufficient time without work in among sessions to keep away from overtraining, which could reason exhaustion, a decline in standard performance, and a higher threat of harm.

five. Mix Up Your Exercises: To save you injuries from repetitive stress, combination up your training routine with distinct physical video video games and techniques.

6. Seek Professional Advice: For individualized steering on exercise strategies, harm prevention, and recuperation strategies, communicate with a expert personal teacher or physiotherapist.

Recovering from an harm and stopping new ones are approximately greater than just retaining off pain—they'll be moreover about engaging in your lengthy-time period fitness goals and improving your overall performance.

Embrace a Holistic Approach to Recovery and Prevention

You also can decorate muscle restoration, avoid injuries, and feature yourself for lengthy-term success in your muscle-constructing endeavors via way of implementing the ones methods into your regimen. Remember, the vital factor to undertaking fantastic physical adjustments is having a robust, healthy body.

Utilizing Supplements for Optimal Muscle Growth

You can reflect onconsideration on using nutritional supplements at the same time as you start your muscle-constructing adventure to boost your exercising and maximize your outcomes. Supplements can deliver a further advantage at the same time as used appropriately, but they can not take the location of a wholesome weight-reduction plan and regular exercising. This bankruptcy can have a take a look at the technology underlying dietary dietary dietary supplements, highlight the excellent options for building muscle, and offer recommendations for a way to make use of them maximum effectively.

Recognizing the Function of Supplements

There is not any magic bullet in phrases of building muscle. They are meant for use along aspect a balanced weight loss plan and prepared workout routine to offer greater nutrients that might useful useful resource in muscle growth, restore, and standard performance.

Essential Supplements for Muscle Growth

1. Protein powder: The constructing blocks of muscular tissue are proteins.

Adequate protein intake is vital for every muscle increase and restore. If you discover it tough to get enough protein from diet by myself, protein powder is probably a available way to up your protein consumption.

2. Creatine: The absolutely taking place chemical called creatine is observed in muscle cells. It can also sell electricity and muscular will growth and beneficial useful resource inside the augmentation of muscle energy production.

three. Branched-Chain Amino Acids (BCAAs): These essential amino acids are involved inside the production of muscle protein and may assist reduce stiffness within the muscles after workout.

4. Fish Oil: Omega-3 fatty acids, which may be decided in fish oil, provide anti-inflammatory characteristics which could accelerate muscle repair and decrease ache.

Suggestions for the Best Supplement Use

1. See a Healthcare professional: To make sure a trendy complement habitual is consistent and suitable for you, see a healthcare expert in advance than beginning it.

2. Select Reputable Brands for High-Quality Supplements: This will guarantee which you are receiving the materials you are finding out to shop for.

three. Adhere to Recommended Doses: To save you any awful results, make sure you're taking nutritional supplements as directed at the labels.

4. The key's timing: plan your supplementation primarily based on your workout routine and specific requirements. To optimize protein synthesis, for example, protein powder can be taken sincerely after exercising.

5. Supplements Don't Replace a Healthy Diet: The key to constructing muscle and retaining large health is a properly-balanced

weight-reduction plan whole of entire, unprocessed elements. A balanced diet plan should be supplemented, not substituted, with supplements.

Recall that supplements cannot replace diligence and determination. The foundations of muscular increase are present day loading, correct shape, and consistency.

Strategically Utilize the Power of Supplements

Supplements can drastically decorate your muscle-building efforts while applied well. To optimize your earnings and acquire your bodily desires, combine them with a nutritious eating regimen, regular exercising, and enough rest. Recall that nutritional supplements aren't achievement guarantees, but rather system to enhance your enjoy.

Chapter 6: Tracking Your Progress and Making Adjustments

To get the frame you want, you have got to expose your progress and make vital adjustments as you begin your muscle-building journey. You might also spot areas for improvement, modify your weight-reduction plan and workout plans hence, and recognize your fulfillment with the resource of maintaining music of your achievements. This economic disaster will cowl a way to song your improvement efficiently and provide recommendation on a way to make facts-pushed modifications to beautify your consequences.

The Importance of Tracking Your Progress

Monitoring your development gives you essential records about your course to gaining muscle, allowing you to:

1. Measure Your Progress: You can display your development in terms of favored body composition, muscular definition, and

strength will increase with the usage of quantitative statistics.

2. Find Your Improvement Areas: You can find out areas wherein you may need to adjust your education, weight loss plan, or recuperation plans through evaluating your development.

3. Remain Motivated: Making improvement inside the path of your goals can be quite energizing on the equal time as you notice it taking location.

4. Make Data-Driven Adjustments: Monitoring your improvement lets in you to decide at the great course of motion for your weight loss plan and schooling with the beneficial useful resource of offering you with the crucial facts.

Effective Methods for Tracking Your Progress

1. Tracking Your Strength Gain: To maintain tabs on your energy development, observe the weights and repetitions you use for every exercise.

2. Body Composition Tracking: Take regular measurements of your waist circumference, body weight, and frame fats % to assess adjustments in your regular frame composition.

three. Visual monitoring: Take pics of your improvement so you can see how your body's shape and muscle definition have modified.

four. Training Logs: Keep tune of all the carrying sports, gadgets, repetitions, weights, and any extra remarks or observations you are making in the direction of your training in a schooling magazine.

five. Nutrition Journals: Maintain a meals magazine to display display screen your day by day consumption and make sure you are becoming enough energy, protein, and carbs to guide muscle constructing.

Making Data-Driven Adjustments

It's time to make changes to maximize your consequences after amassing statistics from tracking your development:

1. Strength Plateaus: If you are not gaining electricity, consider lifting heavier weights, taking fewer breaks, or the usage of extra cutting-edge training techniques.

2. Body Composition Stagnation: Assess your calorie consumption, macronutrient balance, and schooling intensity if your meant modifications in frame composition are not being carried out.

3. Training Plateaus: Try such as new sports activities, converting up your exercise exercises, or adjusting your rest instances if your improvement stops.

four. Nutritional deficits: Give nutrient-dense meals a pinnacle priority and, if wished, consider supplementing in case your nutrients mag indicates any deficits.

five. Recovery Concerns: Give proper sleep and restoration techniques priority, and alter your schooling amount, intensity, and rest durations in case you're feeling worn-out or sore all the time.

Recall that tracking your development is a non-prevent approach in region of an isolated incident.

Accept Constant Improvement and Achieve Your Goals

You can find out your manner to reaching your muscle-constructing dreams through using frequently monitoring your improvement, adjusting based totally mostly on information, and high-quality-tuning your diet plan and exercising ordinary. Recall that increase isn't always linear, but you may exchange your frame and gain new heights of power and fitness in case you are devoted, continual, and flexible.

Setting Realistic Goals and Expectations

It's fantastic to start a muscle-building adventure with ambition and tenacity. Setting less expensive expectancies and goals, but, is crucial to retaining motivation, retaining off discouragement, and making long-term development. This financial ruin will cover techniques for controlling expectancies, organising cheap desires, and making sure your journey is satisfying and excellent.

The Importance of Realistic Goals

Realistic cause-placing has numerous advantages:

1. Achievable Objectives: Realistic goals are to be had and in line with your present degree of fitness, training information, and life-style choices.

2. Sustained Motivation: Reaching low-cost desires offers you top notch reinforcement, which continues you inspired and involved inside the manner.

3. Avoiding Discouragement: Having unrealistic expectancies can purpose you to be upset and discouraged, that would stop you in your tracks.

four. Sustainable Progress: Achieving practical desires lets in everyday, regular improvement that fosters prolonged-term achievement.

Strategies for Setting Realistic Goals

1. Think About Your Starting Point: Determine your cutting-edge energy, frame composition, and diploma of fitness to create viable desires that in shape your functionality.

2. Set SMART desires: Set unique, measurable, conceivable, relevant, and time-positive to ensure your desires are smooth, measurable, and constant together with your time table.

three. Seek Guidance: For individualized steerage on creating practical goals based to your particular dreams and situations, speak with a certified non-public instructor or nutritionist.

four. Break Down Goals into Smaller Steps: To installation a easy path ahead, smash your long-term goals down into smaller, extra feasible obligations.

Controlling Expectations

1. Understand the Process: Acknowledge that developing muscle is a slow tool that requires perseverance, willpower, and a healthy weight-reduction plan.

2. Accept Individuality: Different people development at superb prices for some of reasons, together with genetics, beyond training, and lifestyle selections.

3. Celebrate Little Victories: Regardless of ways minor they will seem, recognize and honor your accomplishments alongside the street.

Chapter 7: Maintaining Motivation and Discipline

Sustaining discipline and motivation is essential to undertaking your muscle-building desires. It's now not generally simple to obtain a sculpted body; there can be times even as region and motivation falter. You may additionally, however, conquer those limitations and continue to be committed to your long-term dreams when you have the correct techniques and mindset. This bankruptcy will cowl practical techniques for preserving disciplined, staying stimulated, and turning your muscle-constructing journey into an extended-time period quest for personal growth.

The Importance of Discipline and Motivation

The topics that preserve you transferring in the route of your desires are location and motivation. They offer you with the inner spark that kindles your enthusiasm, the dedication to preserve going, and the fortitude to transport beyond setbacks.

Techniques for Maintaining Motivation

1. Create a compelling "Why": Link your musculature desires to a more profound purpose that aligns together along with your values and dreams.

2. Visualize Your Success: Regularly, see yourself undertaking your dreams. Conjure up photographs in your thoughts of your modified frame and the feel of pleasure that incorporates success.

3. Seek Inspiration: Be in the enterprise of splendid humans who have succeeded in achieving their fitness objectives. Take idea from their perseverance and provoking memories.

4. Celebrate Milestones: To preserve motivation and provide extraordinary reinforcement, recognize and feature a exquisite time your accomplishments, no matter how minor.

5. Find Pleasure inside the Process: Figure out the way to feature property you

experience for your weight loss plan and workout ordinary.

Cultivating Discipline

1. Establish Routines: To upload form and predictability, establish regular physical games to your exercise, meal guidance, and dozing time desk.

2. Establish Achievable Goals and Manage Expectations: To prevent discouragement and preserve optimism, create feasible goals and manage expectancies.

three. Exercise Self-Discipline: You can exercise energy of thoughts with the aid of manner of manner of being alert, keeping off distractions, and placing your desires ahead of your desires proper away.

four. Seek Accountability: To live devoted and get guide alongside the road, search for an responsibility accomplice or be a part of a fitness community.

five. Accept Challenges: See boundaries as opportunities for personal improvement, use them to provide a lift on your strength of mind, and hone your strategies.

Recall that place and motivation are capabilities that can be reinforced and evolved over the years in choice to ordinary attributes.

Adopt a Growth Mentality to Reach Long-Term Success

Through the improvement of motivation, willpower, and a growth mentality, you can flip your adventure to advantage muscle into an ongoing quest for private development. Recall that success is a chronic system of growth, analyzing, and self-transformation in place of a holiday spot. As you shape your body and turn out to be the greatest model of your self, embody the pains and rejoice in your achievements.

Embracing a Healthy Lifestyle for Long-Term Success

Your course to gaining muscle is ready more than definitely converting your body; it's far approximately adopting a whole outlook on fitness and nicely-being that promotes lengthy-term achievement. You may also optimize your body's regular performance, beautify your highbrow sturdiness, and build an extended-lasting basis for achieving your fitness desires and beyond via embracing wholesome way of life practices. This financial disaster will talk the importance of essential a wholesome way of lifestyles and offer recommendations on the way to comprise these practices into your everyday regular.

The Importance of a Healthy Lifestyle

1. Improved Physical Performance: Maintaining a healthy way of life offers you the power, persistence, and recuperation you want to keep up your wearing sports and get the most out of your muscular increase.

2. Better Mental Well-Being: Stress may be minimized, temper can be improved, and cognitive characteristic can be reinforced with

the assist of proper behavior like normal exercise and sufficient sleep.

three. Decreased Risk of Chronic Illnesses: Living a wholesome lifestyle reduces your hazard of getting continual ailments, that can stop your efforts to get extra in shape and improve your widespread health.

4. Prolonged Life: Adopting healthy behaviors extends one's lifespan and improves one's contemporary state of properly-being.

Strategies for Embracing a Healthy Lifestyle

1. Nourishing Nutrition: Make nice you get sufficient protein, carbs, specific fat, nutrients, and minerals by using way of the use of emphasizing a balanced weight-reduction plan full of entire, unprocessed foods.

2. Frequent Physical Activity: To decorate muscle electricity, cardiovascular fitness, and popular fitness, at the side of as a minimum

half of-hour of moderate-depth interest most days of the week.

three. Sufficient Sleep: To permit your body to heal, regenerate, and be geared up for day after today's sports activities, purpose for 7-8 hours of accurate sleep every night time.

4. Stress manage: To enhance intellectual health and fashionable well-being, engage in stress-discount practices like yoga, meditation, or time spent in nature.

five. Hydration: To keep body functioning, maximize normal performance, and decorate nutrient absorption, drink masses of water finally of the day.

Recall that fundamental a healthful life-style is prepared making regular, high excellent decisions that promote your latest nicely-being in choice to striving for perfection.

Nurturing Well-Being for a Sustainable Fitness Journey

You can also moreover furthermore beautify your famous nicely-being and lay a stable basis on your muscle-building adventure with the useful resource of manner of incorporating the ones wholesome practices into your regular ordinary. Never overlook approximately that dwelling a healthful manner of lifestyles includes greater than truely your bodily makeover. You might also additionally acquire your fitness dreams over the long term and function a more fun existence thru setting your wellknown fitness and properly-being first. Accept the adventure, contend with your frame and mind, and discover how a wholesome way of lifestyles also can change your lifestyles.

Celebrating Your Achievements and Sharing Your Knowledge

You'll hit severa roadblocks and successes along the manner as you develop muscle; they are all symptoms and signs and symptoms of your hard artwork, patience, and unshakable willpower to your goals.

Along the street, you can moreover choose out up insightful expertise and abilties that will help you for your fitness quest and feature an concept to others. This financial disaster will talk the rate of acknowledging and sharing your accomplishments, similarly to accepting the remodeling capability of private improvement and undoubtedly influencing others.

Why It's Important to Celebrate Achievements

No matter how massive or small, celebrating your accomplishments is an crucial part of the journey. It permits you to:

1. Acknowledge Your Progress: Feeling proud of yourself for what you have executed encourages you to keep going after your dreams.

2. Boost Confidence: Acknowledging your accomplishments gives you greater self-self guarantee, which lets in you to tackle new

demanding conditions and obtain even better dreams.

3. Savor the Journey: You may additionally additionally revel in the approach and discover achievement for your health adventure with the aid of acknowledging your victories alongside the way.

four. Motivate Others: Your accomplishments can also act as a catalyst for others to soak up health as a personal task.

Strategies for Celebrating Achievements

1. Reflect on Your Journey: Give your improvement a few concept, noting the worrying conditions you have faced and the competencies you've got got received along the way.

2. Share Your Successes: Let encouraging buddies, own family, or on line groups realise approximately your triumphs so they will be a part of you in celebrating and feeling glad for you.

3. Reward Yourself: Give yourself a substantial cope with or bask in a a laugh hobby to expose yourself how devoted and dedicated you are.

4. Record Your Progress: To see your improvement and apprehend your accomplishments, hold a document of your accomplishments using health trackers, journals, or snap shots.

Sharing Your Knowledge and Impacting Others

Sharing the understanding and knowledge you acquire to your fitness journey with others may additionally have a extraordinary impact:

1. Encouraging Others: By providing your know-how and research, you may encourage others to make well-knowledgeable options regarding their health endeavors.

2. Building a Community of Support: Participating in fitness forums and companies can assist to set up a community of useful

useful resource wherein human beings can grow, research from, and encourage every different.

3. Encouraging Personal Development: You can encourage people to artwork within the course in their personal improvement through sharing your information.

four. Having a Positive Impact: Your recommendation and know-how have the electricity to encourage humans out of doors of your right away social circle to manual higher lives.

Strategies for Sharing Your Knowledge

1. Participate in Online Communities: Share your facts, reply to inquiries, and provide help to others via taking detail in online health boards, businesses, and social media web sites.

2. Provide Educational Content: Give others useful records and direction thru sharing your mind through blog entries, articles, or movement pictures.

three. Provide advise and Support: Provide oldsters that are searching out help and motivation on their health journeys with individualized advise and assist.

four. Lead by the use of Example: Use your development as motivation and often practice healthy conduct to reveal off your statistics and determination.

Remember that the benefits of personal development move past your accomplishments and consist of the have an effect on you may have on unique humans.

Chapter 8: The Science Behind Muscle Building

Building muscle is a reason shared with the resource of the usage of many health enthusiasts and athletes. The approach of muscle building, scientifically called hypertrophy, includes a complex interaction of things that affect muscle growth. By know-how the generation at the back of hypertrophy, human beings can optimize their training and nutrients techniques to obtain the first rate results.

Hypertrophy: An Overview

Hypertrophy refers to the boom in duration of muscle cells, resulting in extra muscle mass and energy. This system happens in reaction to outside stimuli, which incorporates resistance education, which places pressure on the muscle fibers. There are number one kinds of hypertrophy: myofibrillar and sarcoplasmic.

1. Myofibrillar Hypertrophy: This form of hypertrophy includes an increase inside the

tremendous range and length of myofibrils internal muscle fibers. Myofibrils are responsible for muscle contractions, and an boom of their density leads to greater power. Myofibrillar hypertrophy is normally inspired via heavy weightlifting with decrease repetitions.

2. Sarcoplasmic Hypertrophy: Sarcoplasm is the fluid surrounding myofibrils inside muscle cells, containing strength substrates and one-of-a-kind vital additives. Sarcoplasmic hypertrophy entails an growth inside the quantity of sarcoplasm, main to extra muscle endurance and duration. This form of hypertrophy is frequently as a result of higher rep ranges and shorter rest intervals.

Mechanisms of Hypertrophy

Hypertrophy takes place due to a mixture of mechanical anxiety, metabolic stress, and muscle damage. Mechanical anxiety refers back to the force exerted on muscle fibers at some point of resistance schooling. This anxiety stimulates the release of boom factors and activates satellite tv for pc tv for laptop cells, which can be accountable for muscle restore and growth.

Metabolic stress effects from the buildup of metabolites collectively with lactate in the end of immoderate-repetition training. This stress triggers the discharge of hormones like boom hormone and insulin-like growth element 1 (IGF-1), each of which sell muscle boom.

Muscle harm takes vicinity at the same time as muscle fibers experience microtears throughout excessive workout workouts. The frame's restore manner includes satellite tv for pc tv for pc television for pc cells fusing with muscle fibers, essential to an increase in muscle length and strength.

Training Strategies for Hypertrophy

To stimulate hypertrophy efficiently, humans want to interest on incorporating a mixture of training variables:

1. Progressive Overload: Gradually growing the resistance lifted through the years is vital to keep hard muscle agencies and promoting boom.

2. Repetition Ranges: Mixing rep levels, which includes every lower reps with heavier weights and higher reps with slight weights, can target unique kinds of hypertrophy.

3. Rest Intervals: Varying relaxation intervals influences the metabolic pressure on muscle groups. Shorter rests (30-60 seconds) promote sarcoplasmic hypertrophy, on the equal time as longer rests (2-3 mins) opt for myofibrillar hypertrophy.

4. Exercise Selection: Incorporating compound wearing events like squats, deadlifts, and bench presses engages multiple muscle companies, growing a robust stimulus for growth.

Nutrition for Hypertrophy

Proper nutrients plays a pivotal feature in supporting muscle growth:

1. Protein Intake: Consuming ok protein (spherical 1.2 to two.Zero grams in line with kilogram of body weight) materials amino acids essential for muscle restore and increase.

2. Caloric Surplus: To construct muscle, the body calls for a slight caloric surplus, making sure there are sufficient energy and nutrients available for boom.

3. Nutrient Timing: Eating protein and carbohydrates throughout the workout window can resource in muscle healing and pinnacle off glycogen shops.

Understanding the technological information of hypertrophy empowers humans to make informed choices approximately their education and nutrients techniques. By combining right training strategies, contemporary overload, and centered nutrients, anybody can free up their functionality for muscle increase. Remember that consistency, strength of mind, and a holistic technique are key to reaching the extraordinary outcomes on your muscle-constructing adventure.

Effective Nutrition Strategies for Maximal Muscle Growth

Achieving maximal muscle growth involves greater than just lifting weights; right vitamins is a vital component of the equation. By fueling your frame with the proper nutrients on the proper times, you could optimize muscle recovery, repair, and boom. This financial catastrophe will delve into powerful vitamins strategies that useful resource your muscle-building dreams.

The Role of Nutrition in Muscle Growth

Nutrition performs a pivotal function in growing the most appropriate surroundings for muscle growth. When you have interplay in resistance schooling, your muscular tissues undergo stress and microtears. Proper nutrition lets in restore these tears and build new muscle mass, leading to extended muscle length and energy.

Key Nutrition Strategies

1. Protein Intake

Protein is the constructing block of muscle tissues. Adequate protein consumption is important to offer your body with the amino acids required for muscle repair and increase. Aim for a protein consumption of about 1.2 to two.Zero grams of protein in line with kilogram of body weight. High-fine protein assets embody lean meats, hen, fish, eggs, dairy, legumes, and plant-based totally protein dietary dietary supplements.

2. Caloric Surplus

To collect muscle, you need to eat greater energy than you burn (caloric surplus). This gives your body with the power it needs for muscle repair and growth. However, hold in mind of the excess—excessive calorie intake can result in undesirable fat gain.

three. Carbohydrates for Energy

Carbohydrates are your frame's primary deliver of power. They top off glycogen shops in muscle mass, making sure you have got the stamina and power for immoderate exercise workouts. Focus on complex carbohydrates like whole grains, stop end result, and greens for sustained power.

4. Healthy Fats

Healthy fats play a function in hormone production and standard fitness. Incorporate belongings like avocados, nuts, seeds, and fatty fish into your weight-reduction plan. While fats are calorie-dense, they want to no longer be omitted, as they make a contribution for your frame's ordinary nutritional balance.

5. Timing and Nutrient Distribution

Nutrient timing can impact muscle boom. Consume a balanced meal containing protein and carbohydrates interior some hours after your exercise to aid muscle recuperation. Additionally, spacing out your protein consumption within the path of the day can provide a normal deliver of amino acids for muscle restore.

6. Hydration

Staying hydrated is essential for optimum pleasant muscle function and healing. Water lets in shipping nutrients to cells and aids in disposing of waste products. Dehydration can impair performance and avoid muscle increase, so motive to drink masses of water at a few level inside the day.

7. Micronutrients

Vitamins and minerals are vital for numerous physiological techniques, which encompass muscle characteristic. Ensure your diet regime includes quite some nutrient-rich food to satisfy your micronutrient needs. Consider consulting a healthcare professional or registered dietitian to select out any unique deficiencies.

Supplements for Muscle Growth

While entire meals must be your number one source of nutrients, dietary dietary supplements may be used to fill gaps for your weight loss plan. Some normally used nutritional supplements for muscle growth encompass:

1. Whey Protein: Easily digestible and rich in crucial amino acids, whey protein is a convenient preference to meet your protein requirements.

2. Creatine: This supplement can enhance muscle strength and persistence thru developing the provision of power in the course of excessive-depth sports.

three. Branched-Chain Amino Acids (BCAAs): BCAAs can useful aid in muscle recovery and reduce muscle protein breakdown, particularly for the duration of excessive education.

four. Multivitamins: A multivitamin can assist ensure you've got grow to be a balanced intake of essential vitamins and minerals.

Nutrition is a cornerstone of a hit muscle boom. By enforcing effective nutrients techniques, you may provide your body with the vital vitamins to get higher, restore, and bring together muscle. Remember that consistency in every your training and dietary choices is essential to reaching your muscle-building desires. Consult with a healthcare professional or registered dietitian to tailor your vitamins plan on your character desires and optimize your effects.

Chapter 9: The Role of Protein Synthesis

Protein synthesis is a essential organic device that performs a crucial feature in constructing lean muscle agencies. Understanding how protein synthesis works can empower people to make informed choices approximately their weight loss program, exercise, and healing strategies to maximize muscle growth. In this financial ruin, we are going to discover the concept of protein synthesis and its significance in muscle building.

Protein Synthesis: An Overview

Protein synthesis is the way with the resource of using which cells construct new proteins from amino acids. In the context of muscle building, protein synthesis includes the arrival of muscle proteins, which is probably vital for muscle growth, restore, and protection. Two important stages of protein synthesis are transcription and translation:

1. Transcription: In the nucleus of cells, DNA is transcribed into messenger RNA (mRNA). The

mRNA includes the genetic facts vital for protein production.

2. Translation: The mRNA travels to ribosomes, wherein it serves as a template for assembling amino acids into a specific collection. This collection paperwork a trendy protein.

Protein Synthesis and Muscle Growth

Muscle boom takes place whilst the rate of muscle protein synthesis exceeds the rate of muscle protein breakdown. Resistance schooling triggers a chain of activities that sell muscle protein synthesis:

1. Mechanical Tension: Lifting weights creates mechanical anxiety on muscle fibers, main to the activation of satellite tv for pc cells. These cells make contributions to muscle repair and growth.

2. Hormonal Response: Resistance education stimulates the release of hormones like testosterone, increase hormone, and insulin-like boom difficulty 1 (IGF-1). These hormones

promote protein synthesis and muscle increase.

three. Nutrient Availability: Amino acids from dietary protein play a essential role in fueling protein synthesis. Consuming protein-wealthy meals after physical activities gives the building blocks vital for muscle restore and increase.

Maximizing Protein Synthesis

To maximize muscle boom, human beings can undertake techniques that decorate protein synthesis:

1. Protein Timing: Consuming protein-rich food earlier than and after sports can provide amino acids whilst your muscles need them the maximum. This supports muscle restoration and boom.

2. Amino Acid Profile: Different protein resources offer diverse amino acid profiles. Including some of protein property to your weight loss program guarantees you are

getting a numerous style of amino acids for maximum suitable protein synthesis.

three. Leucine-rich Foods: Leucine, an important amino acid, is in particular critical for starting up protein synthesis. Foods rich in leucine include meat, dairy, eggs, and legumes.

four. Progressive Overload: Engaging in contemporary-day resistance schooling annoying conditions muscle corporations and creates the stimulus for protein synthesis. Gradually developing the weight or depth of your exercising workouts is prime.

5. Rest and Recovery: Giving your muscles time to get higher is critical for protein synthesis to occur. Aim for forty eight to seventy hours of restoration time amongst on foot the same muscle enterprise.

6. Sleep Quality: Adequate sleep is critical for hormone law and ordinary recuperation. Aim for 7-9 hours of splendid sleep regular with night time time.

Protein synthesis is a cornerstone of muscle constructing, driving the boom and repair of muscle groups. By statistics the technological knowledge in the back of this way and applying effective strategies, individuals can optimize their muscle-building efforts. Balancing right nutrients, focused exercising, and right enough restoration time will make a contribution to developing an surroundings conducive to protein synthesis and, ultimately, the achievement of lean muscle mass dreams. Remember that consistency and a holistic method are key to successful muscle constructing.

Progressive Overload: Key Principle for Continuous Muscle Development

Progressive overload is a important precept in energy training and muscle building. It includes progressively increasing the needs located to your muscular tissues to stimulate growth and version. By constantly utilising modern-day-day overload, human beings can obtain continuous muscle development and prevent plateaus in their fitness journey. This monetary disaster will delve into the idea of modern overload and the manner to effectively positioned into impact it for your exercising exercises.

Understanding Progressive Overload

Progressive overload refers to the sluggish growth of resistance, intensity, or extent in your workouts through the years. As your muscle agencies adapt to the strain imposed on them, you should little by little project them to hold making earnings. Without this ongoing assignment, your development may stagnate.

The Science Behind Progressive Overload

Muscle increase is a reaction to the pressure and damage due to resistance schooling. When you boost weights, you create microtears in muscle fibers. In the way of recuperation, the body upkeep and strengthens the muscle fibers, maximum vital to muscle growth.

To make sure that this growth keeps, the stimulus have to constantly boom. This is in which revolutionary overload comes into play. By step by step developing the load you growth, the extensive style of repetitions, or the intensity of your workout workout routines, you usually undertaking your muscle organizations, prompting them to comply and increase stronger.

Implementing Progressive Overload

To efficiently put into effect current-day overload, recall the following strategies:

1. Increase Resistance: Gradually boom the burden you bring for each exercise. For instance, if you're squatting 50 kg this week, aim for fifty .Five kg next week.

2. Adjust Repetitions and Sets: Increase the variety of repetitions or gadgets you perform for a given exercise. For instance, if you're doing 3 devices of eight reps, strive 4 devices of 8 reps.

three. Manipulate Intensity: Alter the depth of your physical activities with the aid of the usage of reducing rest intervals amongst gadgets or incorporating strategies like drop devices or supersets.

4. Vary Exercises: Introduce new wearing sports activities that focus on the equal muscle businesses from fantastic angles. This challenges your muscular tissues in novel techniques and prevents version.

five. Track Progress: Keep a exercising magazine or use a health app to record your lifts, repetitions, and units. Tracking your development allows you display your improvements and regulate your exercising sports for that reason.

Chapter 10: Optimizing Recovery for Faster Muscle Growth

Optimal restoration is a essential but frequently left out thing of muscle constructing. While excessive sporting activities stimulate muscle increase, it's far for the duration of the healing phase that actual restore and growth stand up. By adopting effective healing strategies, humans can accelerate the muscle-building technique, reduce the danger of harm, and decorate commonplace normal usual performance. In this bankruptcy, we're going to find out techniques to optimize restoration for quicker muscle boom and repair.

Understanding Recovery in Muscle Building

Recovery involves permitting your body to heal, restore, and adapt after excessive bodily hobby. During workout workouts, muscle fibers go through stress and microtears. Proper healing guarantees the ones tears are repaired and results in muscle increase. Ignoring restoration can result in overtraining, reduced overall performance, and increased hazard of damage.

Key Recovery Strategies

1. Quality Sleep

Sleep is one of the maximum vital components of healing. During deep sleep ranges, the body releases increase hormone, which aids in muscle repair and boom. Aim for 7-nine hours of uninterrupted sleep each night time time time to aid top of the line recuperation.

2. Nutrition and Hydration

Proper nutrients is vital for muscle restore and growth. Focus on ingesting a balanced diet plan with good enough protein, carbohydrates, and wholesome fat. Hydration is similarly crucial, as water helps nutrient delivery and waste removal.

3. Active Recovery

Engaging in slight, low-depth sports at the side of taking walks, cycling, or yoga on rest days can enhance blood pass and help flush out metabolic waste from muscle tissues, assisting in restoration.

4. Foam Rolling and Stretching

Using a foam roller can help release muscle tension and decorate flexibility. Incorporating dynamic and static stretching can also enhance blood drift, reduce muscle stiffness, and enhance regular form of movement.

five. Cold and Heat Therapy

Alternating between ice and warmth remedies can reduce contamination and promote blood drift, assisting in restoration. Ice can help with acute pain and contamination, on the same time as warmness can loosen up muscle groups and decorate movement.

6. Massage and Myofascial Release

Massage remedy and myofascial launch strategies can alleviate muscle ache, decorate blood circulate, and beautify recuperation.

Consider everyday massages or using tools like rub down sticks or foam rollers.

7. Stress Management

High stages of strain can negatively effect restoration and not unusual health. Incorporate stress-good deal strategies consisting of meditation, deep breathing, and mindfulness to assist your frame's recuperation techniques.

eight. Proper Warm-up and Cool-down

Effective warm-up routines boom blood flow, beautify joint mobility, and put together muscle groups for the approaching exercising. A thorough cool-down allows lessen positioned up-exercise muscle pain and supports restoration.

nine. Listen to Your Body

Pay hobby to signs of overtraining, fatigue, or lingering muscle ache. Rest at the same time as desired and keep away from pushing your frame past its limits, as this may prevent recuperation and development.

10. Rest Days

Scheduled rest days are essential for restoration. They offer your muscle groups time to repair and adapt, stopping burnout and overtraining. Use relaxation days to recognition on recuperation techniques like stretching, foam rolling, and relaxation.

Optimizing healing is a essential factor of a success muscle building. Without proper recuperation, the body can't repair and broaden muscles effectively. By imposing techniques together with outstanding sleep, proper vitamins, active healing, and pressure manipulate, you can manual your body's natural recuperation techniques and accelerate muscle growth. Remember that recovery is not a one-period-suits-all technique—be aware of your body, modify your techniques as wished, and prioritize every education and recovery for sustainable muscle-building success.

Balancing Cardio and Weightlifting for Lean Muscle Building

Balancing cardiovascular exercising and weightlifting is a not unusual undertaking for individuals looking for lean muscle development. While weightlifting is essential for constructing muscle, cardiovascular sporting activities offer their private set of blessings. Striking the proper balance a number of the two will will can help you gather a lean, muscular frame at the equal time as maintaining cardiovascular fitness. This monetary catastrophe explores the manner to mix each varieties of exercising successfully for most suitable outcomes.

The Role of Weightlifting in Muscle Building

Weightlifting, additionally called resistance training, is a cornerstone of muscle development. It involves lifting weights to create tension on your muscle organizations, leading to microtears that the body upkeep and strengthens. Over time, this manner results in muscle growth and prolonged energy.

Key advantages of weightlifting for muscle constructing encompass:

1. Increased Muscle Mass: Resistance training stimulates muscle protein synthesis, leading to muscle boom and definition.

2. Enhanced Strength: Lifting weights little by little disturbing conditions muscle mass, vital to increased electricity and strength.

three. Metabolic Boost: Muscle tissue burns extra energy at relaxation than fats tissue, contributing to advanced metabolism.

4. Bone Health: Weightlifting permits increase bone density, decreasing the danger of osteoporosis.

The Role of Cardiovascular Exercise

Cardiovascular workout, often called aerobic, focuses on improving cardiovascular fitness and staying power. This type of exercise engages the heart, lungs, and circulatory device, essential to numerous fitness benefits.

Key blessings of cardiovascular workout consist of:

1. Heart Health: Cardiovascular exercising workouts improve coronary coronary heart fitness thru way of strengthening the coronary coronary heart muscle and enhancing blood go with the waft.

2. Fat Loss: Cardio burns power and may contribute to fats loss at the same time as mixed with a balanced healthy dietweight-reduction plan.

three. Endurance: Cardio improves stamina and staying power, allowing you to interact in longer and similarly immoderate workout routines.

4. Mood Enhancement: Cardio releases endorphins, that might decorate mood and decrease strain.

Balancing Cardio and Weightlifting

Achieving a balance among cardiovascular exercise and weightlifting is important for reaching a lean, muscular body without sacrificing cardiovascular fitness. Here's the way to strike that balance efficaciously:

1. Set Clear Goals: Define your desires—whether they may be muscle boom, fats loss, or common health. This will help you tailor your exercise ordinary for this reason.

2. Prioritize Weightlifting: If your number one aim is building lean muscle, prioritize weightlifting lessons. Aim for three-four electricity training durations in step with week, that specialize in compound bodily video games that engage multiple muscle organizations.

three. Schedule Cardio Strategically: Incorporate aerobic wearing activities on non-weightlifting days or after weightlifting durations. This prevents aerobic from interfering with muscle recovery.

4. Choose the Right Cardio: Opt for mild-intensity aerobic like brisk walking, walking, biking, or swimming. High-intensity c language training (HIIT) moreover can be powerful for burning electricity and improving cardiovascular health.

5. Monitor Intensity and Volume: Pay interest to the intensity and period of each your weightlifting and cardio workout routines. Avoid excessive cardio that would likely save you muscle boom.

6. Adjust Nutrition: Adjust your vitamins based totally to your exercise ordinary. On weightlifting days, make certain you're eating sufficient protein and energy to aid muscle recovery. On cardio days, popularity on staying hydrated and refueling with nutrient-dense meals.

7. Listen to Your Body: If you sense fatigued or overtrained, it's miles crucial to pay attention to your body and prioritize relaxation or active recovery in preference to excessive aerobic.

eight. Plan Periodization: Incorporate periodization into your schooling plan, which includes numerous the depth and quantity of each weightlifting and aerobic over time. This prevents plateaus and allows for proper restoration.

Balancing cardiovascular exercising and weightlifting is vital for undertaking a lean, muscular body whilst preserving cardiovascular fitness. By placing smooth goals, strategically scheduling exercising routines, and adjusting your nutrients, you may successfully combine each types of workout into your routine. Remember that locating the proper balance also can require some trial and errors, so be affected person and adaptable as you refine your approach. Ultimately, a properly-balanced exercising recurring will assist your muscle-building efforts on the same time as selling normal fitness and properly-being.

Tailoring Workouts for Different Body Types: Ectomorph, Mesomorph, Endomorph

When it involves building muscle and venture health dreams, knowledge your body kind can be pretty beneficial. Ectomorphs, mesomorphs, and endomorphs are three first rate body kinds, each with its personal developments and worries. By tailoring your exercising and vitamins strategies for your frame kind, you could optimize your effects and artwork collectively at the side of your natural inclinations. In this bankruptcy, we will discover a manner to layout bodily sports for every body kind: ectomorph, mesomorph, and endomorph.

Ectomorph: The "Hard Gainer"

Ectomorphs will be inclined to have a lean and narrow collect with fast metabolisms. Gaining muscle and weight can be hard for them. To correctly construct muscle as an ectomorph, maintain in mind the subsequent techniques:

1. Focus on Progressive Overload: Prioritize resistance education with a focus on compound sports activities activities that

have interaction multiple muscle businesses. Gradually growth the weight and depth to stimulate muscle growth.

2. Higher Caloric Intake: Ectomorphs frequently have excessive metabolisms, so that they want to consume more calories than they burn to assist muscle increase. Opt for nutrient-dense additives with a balance of protein, carbohydrates, and healthful fats.

3. Frequent Meals: Split your each day caloric intake into numerous small meals to provide a steady deliver of vitamins for muscle repair and boom.

4. Adequate Protein Intake: Consume sufficient protein to assist muscle recovery and boom. Aim for spherical 1.2 to 2.Zero grams of protein in keeping with kilogram of body weight.

Mesomorph: The "Naturally Muscular"

Mesomorphs are virtually muscular and will be inclined to gain muscle groups surprisingly consequences. They actually have a balanced metabolism. To make the maximum in their body type, mesomorphs can observe the ones guidelines:

1. Embrace Variety: Mesomorphs can enjoy an entire lot of exercising styles, such as each electricity education and cardiovascular workout. This flexibility lets in them to preserve muscle whilst staying lean.

2. Balanced Nutrition: Maintain a balanced food regimen with a mild caloric intake. Focus on entire meals and screen detail sizes to keep away from immoderate weight advantage.

three. Monitor Body Composition: Since mesomorphs can advantage muscle and fats without trouble, it is important to reveal body composition to save you excess weight advantage.

four. Combine Cardio and Strength: Incorporate each aerobic and power schooling for a properly-rounded approach. This can help mesomorphs maintain their muscular body even as selling cardiovascular health.

Endomorph: The "Naturally Curvy"

Endomorphs have a tendency to have a simply curvy or stocky construct and might have a slower metabolism, making them more prone to weight gain. To accumulate muscle improvement and control weight effectively, endomorphs can observe those recommendations:

1. Focus on Resistance Training: Prioritize resistance schooling to assemble muscle and improve metabolism. Include compound actions and full-body workout sporting events.

2. Manage Caloric Intake: While electricity are critical for muscle boom, endomorphs want to don't forget of their caloric intake to keep away from extra fats benefit. Consume slightly fewer energy than you burn to promote fats loss.

3. Include Cardio: Incorporate everyday cardiovascular workout to beautify calorie burning and useful useful resource weight manipulate.

four. Choose Nutrient-Dense Foods: Opt for nutrient-dense materials that provide essential vitamins with out extra power. Focus on lean proteins, entire grains, give up end result, and vegetables.

5. Interval Training: Consider excessive-intensity c programming language training (HIIT) for cardio intervals. HIIT can beautify metabolism and promote fats loss in a shorter duration.

Understanding your body type is a precious device for tailoring your physical games and nutrients strategies to maximise outcomes. Whether you're an ectomorph, mesomorph, or endomorph, embracing your herbal tendencies and making informed alternatives permit you to achieve your fitness goals. Keep in thoughts that everyone is particular, and individual elements moreover play a function in how your frame responds to education and vitamins. Consulting with a health professional or registered dietitian can offer customized steering to help you make the most of your frame type and gain your favored outcomes.

Chapter 11: Avoiding Common Mistakes

Building muscle calls for power of thoughts, proper planning, and a solid statistics of effective training and nutrients techniques. However, there are numerous commonplace mistakes that people frequently make on their muscle-building journey that might restriction development and consequences. In this economic break, we're going to highlight the pinnacle 10 muscle-constructing pitfalls to avoid, ensuring that your efforts yield the remarkable possible consequences.

1. Neglecting Proper Form

One of the maximum commonplace mistakes is using fallacious shape during bodily games. Poor form not most effective reduces the effectiveness of the exercising however may even increase the chance of harm. Prioritize analyzing proper technique and lifting with control.

2. Ignoring Warm-up and Cool-down

Skipping heat-up and cool-down carrying activities can result in muscle strains, stiffness, and decreased universal overall performance. Incorporate dynamic stretches and mobility sporting sports earlier than workouts, and devote time to static stretches after to sell flexibility and recuperation.

three. Overtraining

Training too often or without enough relaxation can result in overtraining, which hinders muscle restoration and increase. Allow muscle organizations time to get better among workout routines and listen to your frame's signs of fatigue.

4. Underestimating Nutrition

Nutrition is important for muscle building. Neglecting good enough protein consumption, ingesting bad-awesome materials, and no longer taking note of caloric dreams can all avoid progress. Prioritize a balanced weight loss program with enough protein, carbohydrates, and healthy fat.

5. Not Enough Sleep

Sleep is critical for muscle restoration and ordinary fitness. Aim for 7-9 hours of first rate sleep regular with night time to manual muscle increase, hormone regulation, and cognitive feature.

6. Relying Too Heavily on Supplements

Supplements can play a characteristic in muscle building, but they should complement a balanced weight loss program, no longer replace it. Relying sincerely on dietary nutritional dietary supplements without addressing your simple nutrients can motive suboptimal consequences.

7. Lack of Progression

Sticking to the equal weight and workout routine for too lengthy can purpose a plateau in muscle increase. Incorporate modern overload via grade by grade developing weight, depth, or repetitions to preserve hard your muscle groups.

eight. Neglecting Cardiovascular Health

While muscle constructing is a subject, cardiovascular fitness must not be not noted. Incorporate normal cardiovascular exercise to preserve coronary coronary heart health, staying strength, and widespread fitness.

nine. Focusing on Isolation Exercises

Isolation physical games goal specific muscle agencies, but compound sports activities sports engage more than one muscle groups simultaneously. Prioritize compound actions like squats, deadlifts, and bench presses to stimulate hooked up muscle boom.

10. Impatience

Building muscle takes time and consistency. Expecting in a single day results can result in frustration and discouragement. Stay affected man or woman, live regular, and remember the device.

Avoiding the ones commonplace muscle-constructing pitfalls can notably beautify your development and help to procure your health dreams extra correctly. By prioritizing proper shape, taking note of vitamins and sleep, avoiding overtraining, and embracing a balanced approach to each strength and cardiovascular schooling, you could optimize your muscle-building journey. Remember that constructing muscle is a slow method that calls for determination, patience, and a dedication to common fitness and nicely being. Consulting with fitness experts or registered dietitians can offer personalized guidance and help on your muscle-constructing journey.

The Importance of Sleep in Muscle Recovery and Growth

Sleep is regularly called the "mystery weapon" of muscle recuperation and boom. While vitamins and exercise are vital components of constructing muscle, sleep plays a vital position in optimizing the ones methods. In this economic catastrophe, we are able to find out the essential importance of sleep in muscle recuperation and growth and provide pointers on the way to beautify the amazing of your sleep for higher outcomes.

The Role of Sleep in Muscle Recovery

During sleep, the frame enters severa levels of restorative methods, which incorporates muscle restoration. Here's how sleep contributes to muscle recuperation:

1. Muscle Repair: During deep sleep stages, increase hormone is released, selling muscle restore and healing from the stress of resistance education.

2. Protein Synthesis: Sleep enhances protein synthesis, the process by means of which the frame builds new muscle mass. This allows muscle boom and version.

3. Glycogen Restoration: Sleep allows pinnacle off glycogen shops in muscle companies, providing strength to your next exercising.

4. Inflammation Reduction: Quality sleep reduces irritation, that could stand up because of immoderate exercise. Lower infection levels make contributions to faster recovery.

The Connection Between Sleep and Hormones

Hormones play a vital function in muscle restoration and increase, and sleep has a right away effect on hormone production:

1. Growth Hormone: Deep sleep ranges, in particular the number one few hours of sleep, result in prolonged increase hormone launch. This hormone is vital for muscle restore and growth.

2. Testosterone: Sleep deprivation can bring about decreased testosterone tiers, which can be vital for muscle development, energy, and widespread nicely-being.

3. Cortisol Regulation: Proper sleep permits regulate cortisol, a pressure hormone. Elevated cortisol ranges because of terrible

sleep can avoid muscle restoration and increase.

Practical Tips to Enhance Sleep Quality

To optimize muscle healing and growth, attention on enhancing your sleep exceptional:

1. Consistent Sleep Schedule: Aim to go to mattress and wake up at the identical time every day, even on weekends. Consistency reinforces your frame's internal clock.

2. Create a Restful Environment: Keep your bedroom darkish, quiet, and funky to create an maximum inexperienced sleep surroundings. Consider using blackout curtains and white noise machines if essential.

three. Limit Screen Time: Blue moderate from monitors can intrude with the producing of melatonin, a hormone that regulates sleep. Limit show show publicity an hour in advance than bedtime.

4. Establish a Bedtime Routine: Engage in enjoyable sports activities earlier than mattress, which includes studying, stretching, or deep respiratory, to signal your frame that it is time to wind down.

five. Limit Caffeine and Alcohol: Avoid caffeine and alcohol close to bedtime, as they will be capable of disrupt sleep patterns and prevent the first-class of your rest.

6. Watch Your Diet: Heavy meals and noticeably spiced foods earlier than mattress can motive pain and disrupted sleep. Opt for moderate, balanced snacks if desired.

7. Manage Stress: Practicing strain-discount strategies like meditation, yoga, or deep respiratory can help calm your thoughts in advance than sleep.

eight. Limit Naps: While short electricity naps may be beneficial, extended naps at some stage in the day can intervene with midnight sleep. Aim for naps of 20-half of-hour if desired.

nine. Stay Active: Regular physical hobby can promote higher sleep extraordinary, however avoid immoderate sports activities near bedtime, as they'll be stimulating.

10. Seek Professional Help: If you typically conflict with sleep, keep in mind consulting a healthcare professional to cope with any underlying sleep problems.

Sleep is a cornerstone of powerful muscle recovery and boom. Prioritizing sleep tremendous, preserving a constant sleep time table, and adopting healthy sleep conduct can substantially decorate your muscle-building efforts. Remember that sleep isn't always a passive hobby—it's miles an energetic manner that contributes to your general well-being. By taking steps to beautify your sleep, you can now not splendid see enhancements in muscle recovery and increase however furthermore experience higher standard health and power.

Building Muscle at Home: Effective Tips and Workouts

Building muscle might not continually require a gymnasium membership or access to heavy weights. With the right techniques and creativity, you could efficaciously build muscle in the comfort of your home. Whether you are constrained thru location, gadget, or in reality decide upon the advantage of home exercises, this monetary catastrophe gives powerful guidelines and workout thoughts for constructing muscle at domestic.

Tips for Building Muscle at Home

1. Bodyweight Exercises: Bodyweight bodily activities are a awesome manner to collect muscle without any gadget. Push-ups, squats, lunges, and planks have interaction severa muscle organizations and sell energy development.

2. Use Resistance Bands: Resistance bands are bendy and price-powerful tools which can upload resistance in your exercising workouts. They are to be had in one in each of a type stages of resistance, allowing you to regularly boom the challenge.

3. Incorporate Isometric Holds: Isometric physical video games include retaining a role with out movement, activating muscle groups and constructing strength. Examples encompass wall sits and planks.

four. Get Creative with Household Items: Everyday devices like water jugs, backpacks packed with books, or chairs can function makeshift weights for resistance carrying events.

5. Focus on Form: Proper shape is important to save you damage and efficaciously goal the intended muscle mass. Study films or tutorials to ensure you're performing bodily activities effectively.

6. Progressive Overload: Gradually boom the depth of your sports by way of the use of developing repetitions, gadgets, or resistance. This principle applies to home physical games simply as it does in a gym putting.

7. Prioritize Compound Movements: Compound wearing occasions engage a

couple of muscle groups, imparting a entire exercise. Squats, push-ups, pull-ups (if you have a bar), and dips are great alternatives.

8. Create a Routine: Consistency is important. Develop a workout ordinary that includes numerous sports activities sports and targets wonderful muscle organizations on different days.

Effective Home Workouts for Muscle Building

1. Full-Body Circuit Workout

Perform every exercise for forty five seconds, located with the beneficial resource of 15 seconds of rest. Complete all physical games, rest for 1-2 mins, and repeat for three-four rounds.

Chapter 12: Muscle Mass Building

Understanding the significance of muscular tissues

Muscle mass, furthermore known as lean body mass or muscle groups, refers to the amount of muscle inside the body. It performs a important function in our regular fitness and properly-being. While many human beings associate muscle tissues with aesthetics and bodybuilding, its importance extends an extended manner beyond really appearance.

Metabolism and Weight Management:

Muscle tissue is metabolically energetic, which means it calls for strength (energy) to feature. Having a higher muscle groups will boom your basal metabolic charge (BMR), this is the massive form of energy your frame desires at rest. This technique that people with extra muscular tissues burn more strength even when theyre now not actively exercising. As a prevent end result, keeping or growing muscles can make a contribution to weight control and make it less difficult to keep a wholesome body weight.

Strength and Functional Abilities:

Muscle mass is right away linked to strength and physical performance. Building and retaining muscle thru resistance training permits enhance muscular power, it's critical for wearing out every day sports activities sports, together with lifting gadgets, mountain climbing stairs, or acting manual labour. Strong muscle tissue furthermore makes contributions to higher stability, stability, and coordination, decreasing the risk of falls and injuries, specifically in older adults.

Bone Health:

Having good enough muscle groups is essential for super bone fitness. The strain located on bones within the direction of resistance physical sports stimulates bone increase and could increase bone density, decreasing the hazard of osteoporosis and fractures. Additionally, muscle contractions exert mechanical forces on bones, which permits to hold their power and integrity.

Glucose Regulation and Insulin Sensitivity:

Muscle tissue performs a pivotal function in glucose metabolism. During workout, muscle mass utilise glucose for energy, helping to alter blood sugar stages. Having higher muscle tissues enhances the bodys capacity to keep and utilise glucose, enhancing insulin sensitivity. This can be useful in stopping or coping with situations like kind 2 diabetes.

Hormonal Balance:

Muscle mass influences hormone production and law in the frame. Resistance education stimulates the discharge of increase hormone and testosterone, both of which is probably essential for muscle increase and repair. Adequate muscle groups moreover lets in stability hormones like cortisol, which could have horrific effects at the body while extended for prolonged periods. Hormonal balance is critical for common health, energy, and preserving a wholesome body composition.

Aging and Longevity:

As we age, we certainly enjoy a decline in muscle businesses, known as sarcopenia. This lack of muscle groups and energy can purpose reduced mobility, useful obstacles, and an extended hazard of falls and fractures. However, engaging in regular resistance schooling and retaining muscle companies can assist fight the effects of having vintage, maintain physical characteristic, and enhance sturdiness.

Psychological Well-being:

The advantages of muscle groups increase beyond bodily health. Engaging in electricity schooling and building muscle can also have excessive first rate outcomes on highbrow and emotional nicely-being. Exercise releases endorphins, which can be natural mood enhancers, and can reduce symptoms and signs and symptoms of depression and anxiety. Additionally, attaining personal health goals and experiencing improvements in power and frame can boom self-confidence, vanity, and body photograph.

Setting realistic desires for muscle constructing

Setting realistic desires for muscle constructing is essential for conducting prolonged-time period fulfillment and retaining motivation during your health adventure. Many humans make the mistake of placing unrealistic goals which might be hard to gain, main to frustration and in the end giving up. By putting sensible desires, you can boom a centered and sustainable technique to muscle building that maximises your development even as preserving you endorsed and engaged.

Chapter 13: Anatomy and Physiology

Understanding muscle fibres and brands

Muscle fibres are the character cells that make up our muscle tissues. These fibres play a vital feature in muscle characteristic, energy, and endurance. There are three primary varieties of muscle fibres: Type I (sluggish-twitch), Type IIa (rapid-twitch oxidative), and Type IIb (rapid-twitch glycolytic). Each kind has fantastic tendencies and capabilities, and knowledge them can help optimise schooling techniques for specific goals.

Type I (Slow-Twitch) Muscle Fibres:

Type I muscle fibres are regularly referred to as sluggish-twitch fibres. They are characterized through their immoderate resistance to fatigue and their capacity to preserve contractions over longer durations. These fibres are wealthy in mitochondria, which allows them to generate electricity thru cardio metabolism the usage of oxygen. Type I fibres are splendid proper for staying power sports, along with prolonged-distance strolling or biking.

Key tendencies of Type I muscle fibres:

High persistence and fatigue resistance

Rich in mitochondria for aerobic energy production

Smaller in length in comparison to distinct fibre types

Lower strain production capability in evaluation to rapid-twitch fibres

Red in color due to myoglobin content material

Training for Type I muscle fibres:

To optimise Type I muscle fibres, staying strength training strategies are commonly hired. This includes sports collectively with prolonged-distance walking, cycling, swimming, and exclusive cardio sports that contain sustained, repetitive contractions over prolonged durations. High-repetition, low-intensity resistance education can also stimulate Type I fibres and enhance their staying power capability.

Type IIa (Fast-Twitch Oxidative) Muscle Fibres:

Type IIa muscle fibres are taken into consideration intermediate fibres, combining traits of each gradual-twitch and speedy-twitch fibres. They own a distinctly excessive resistance to fatigue and a mild functionality for pressure manufacturing. Type IIa fibres have a better aerobic capacity than Type IIb fibres however although depend upon anaerobic metabolism to a big quantity. These fibres are involved in sports activities that require each staying energy and energy, which consist of middle-distance going for walks or swimming.

Key trends of Type IIa muscle fibres:

Moderate persistence and fatigue resistance

Can generate power through each aerobic and anaerobic metabolism

Intermediate in length between Type I and Type IIb fibres

Greater stress production functionality in assessment to Type I fibres

Pinkish-pink in shade due to myoglobin content material

Training for Type IIa muscle fibres:

Training techniques that concentrate on Type IIa fibres contain a combination of moderate-intensity staying electricity physical games and power schooling. This consists of sports activities like interval education, tempo runs, circuit education, and mild-load resistance training with mild repetitions. By stimulating each cardio and anaerobic power systems, Type IIa fibres may be optimised for each staying strength and electricity.

Type IIb (Fast-Twitch Glycolytic) Muscle Fibres:

Type IIb muscle fibres, additionally known as rapid-twitch fibres, are characterized via the use of their rapid stress manufacturing and excessive capability for anaerobic metabolism. These fibres fatigue quick however have the terrific capability for pressure technology. Type IIb fibres rely on glycogen saved within the muscle for electricity and are in general worried in explosive, immoderate-intensity sports, consisting of sprinting, powerlifting, and leaping.

Key tendencies of Type IIb muscle fibres:

Low staying power and fatigue short

Reliance on anaerobic metabolism for strength manufacturing

Largest in length among muscle fibre kinds

Highest strain manufacturing functionality

White in colour because of decrease myoglobin content material

Training for Type IIb muscle fibres:

To optimise Type IIb muscle fibres, excessive-depth, explosive sports activities sports are important. This includes sports activities like sprinting, heavy weightlifting, plyometrics, and particular power-based moves. Training strategies have to recognition on stimulating the bodys anaerobic strength systems to enhance stress production and power output.

Muscle Fiber Adaptation:

Its vital to have a look at that muscle fibres have the capability to conform to wonderful varieties of training stimuli. Through right education and conditioning, the traits of muscle fibres can shift to better in shape the needs positioned upon them. This is called fibre-type plasticity. While an individuals genetic predisposition determines the distribution of fibre sorts, education can in spite of the reality that result in upgrades in muscle fibre characteristic and universal general performance.

How muscular tissues develop and adapt

Muscle increase and version, furthermore known as muscle hypertrophy, is a complicated physiological approach that happens in response to resistance education or exercising. When muscle mass are subjected to trendy overload, they go through a sequence of structural and beneficial modifications that result in an growth in muscle period, energy, and persistence. Understanding how muscle organizations grow and adapt can help human beings optimise their training carrying activities and acquire their fitness goals.

Muscle fibres, the man or woman cells that make up muscle tissues, are the primary components responsible for muscle growth and version. There are essential kinds of muscle fibres: gradual-twitch (Type I) and speedy-twitch (Type II) fibres. Slow-twitch fibres are greater proof against fatigue and are typically involved in staying energy sports, at the identical time as speedy-twitch fibres generate greater strain however fatigue more rapid and are important for strength and strength sports sports.

When muscles are subjected to resistance education, numerous mechanisms come into play to promote muscle increase and edition:

Mechanical anxiety: Resistance schooling places mechanical stress on the muscle fibres, inflicting microscopic damage to the muscle fibres. This damage triggers a response from the body to restore and make stronger the muscle fibres, primary to muscle growth. Mechanical anxiety can be generated thru numerous wearing sports activities, on the aspect of weightlifting, body weight bodily games, or resistance machines.

Muscle damage: The microscopic damage on account of resistance education turns on satellite tv for pc cells, which can be dormant cells located spherical muscle fibres. These satellite tv for computer cells play a vital role in muscle restore and increase. Upon activation, satellite tv for computer cells fuse to the triumphing muscle fibres, donating their nuclei and other cell additives, thereby selling muscle protein synthesis and facilitating muscle growth.

Metabolic strain: Resistance schooling moreover outcomes in metabolic strain inside the muscle. During exercising, the muscle groups utilise electricity property consisting of adenosine triphosphate (ATP) and glycogen. As the ones energy stores are depleted, metabolic byproducts alongside side lactate, hydrogen ions, and reactive oxygen species gather. This metabolic strain triggers anabolic signalling pathways, selling muscle version.

Hormonal response: Hormones play a vital function in muscle increase and version. Resistance education stimulates the release of anabolic hormones collectively with testosterone, growth hormone, and insulin-like boom element 1 (IGF-1). These hormones decorate muscle protein synthesis, promote tissue restore, and facilitate muscle growth.

Once these mechanisms are added about, muscle increase and variation upward thrust up through a way known as muscle protein synthesis. Muscle protein synthesis is the advent of recent muscle proteins to repair and give a lift to the damaged muscle fibres. It includes the assembly of amino acids, the building blocks of proteins, into complex muscle proteins.

Protein synthesis expenses boom in reaction to resistance training and stay superior for as masses as 48 hours after exercising. Adequate protein intake is important to provide the crucial amino acids for muscle protein synthesis. Consuming protein-wealthy meals or dietary dietary supplements following workout can help optimise muscle increase and variant.

Its important to have a look at that muscle growth isn't always completely determined via the usage of exercising. Factors which includes vitamins, rest, and genetics moreover have an impact at the quantity and fee of muscle boom. A properly-balanced weight-reduction plan that includes an suitable sufficient quantity of protein, carbohydrates, and healthy fats is essential to useful resource muscle growth. Sufficient rest and recovery durations among exercises allow the frame to repair and rebuild muscles.

Furthermore, genetic factors could have an impact on an humans reaction to resistance schooling. Some human beings also can have a genetic predisposition to more muscle growth and version in contrast to others. However, regardless of genetics, constant and modern resistance education coupled with appropriate vitamins and healing can reason terrific muscle boom and model in maximum people.

The characteristic of hormones in muscle building

The role of hormones in muscle building is large and complex. Hormones are chemical messengers that play a vital feature in numerous physiological techniques, along facet muscle growth and improvement. They adjust the synthesis and breakdown of proteins, the building blocks of muscular tissues, and feature an impact on muscular tissues, strength, and regular body composition.

Several hormones have been diagnosed as key players in muscle building, with every hormone exerting unique results on muscle businesses. Lets delve into a number of the essential hormones involved in muscle boom and recognize their roles:

Testosterone: Testosterone is the number one male intercourse hormone and is vital for muscle constructing. It promotes protein synthesis, will growth muscle fibre length, and complements muscle energy. Testosterone moreover stimulates the release of boom hormone and insulin-like increase component-1 (IGF-1), both of which might be crucial for muscle boom.

Chapter 14: Designing Your Training Program

Assessing your contemporary-day fitness diploma

Assessing your present day-day fitness degree is an important step inside the route of expertise your regular health and determining the appropriate exercising and schooling software for your individual needs. Fitness checks provide precious records approximately your strength, staying strength, flexibility, and cardiovascular fitness. By evaluating the ones components, you can set up a baseline and tune your improvement as you figure towards achieving your health desires.

There are numerous key areas to consider even as assessing your contemporary-day health diploma:

Cardiovascular Endurance: Cardiovascular persistence refers to the functionality of your coronary coronary heart, lungs, and blood vessels to supply oxygen to your muscle groups for the duration of sustained physical hobby. Common checks to evaluate cardiovascular staying electricity embody the 1-mile run, three-minute step take a look at, or the beep check. These checks diploma how successfully your frame can utilise oxygen and provide an example of your essential cardiovascular health.

Muscular Strength: Muscular power refers back to the maximum amount of strain your muscle agencies can generate. It is classified through carrying activities like bench press, squats, or deadlifts, in which you deliver frequently heavier weights. You also can use frame weight carrying activities along with push-usaor pull-u.S.A.To gauge your electricity degree. Assessing your muscular energy enables determine the proper weight and resistance to your electricity training software program.

Muscular Endurance: Muscular persistence is the capability of your muscle tissues to carry out repetitive contractions over an prolonged period. Tests for muscular endurance also can encompass carrying activities which includes push-ups, sit down down down-ups, or plank holds. These exams compare how lengthy you can preserve the exercise or how many repetitions you can complete in advance than accomplishing fatigue. Muscular persistence is important for sports activities activities requiring repetitive movements, which encompass jogging or cycling.

Flexibility: Flexibility refers back to the fashion of motion round your joints. It is classified the usage of diverse stretching bodily video video games that target essential muscle groups, including the hamstrings, shoulders, and hips. Tests just like the take a seat down-and-attain check degree the energy of your lower again and hamstrings. Adequate flexibility reduces the chance of injuries and allows for higher normal overall performance in sports sports that require a massive range of motion.

Body Composition: Body composition evaluation evaluates the share of fats, muscle, and distinctive tissues for your body. Common techniques consist of frame mass index (BMI) calculations, skinfold measurements, or superior strategies like twin-electricity X-ray absorptiometry (DEXA) scans. Understanding your frame composition enables decide when you have a healthy weight and if you want to recognition on decreasing frame fats or constructing lean muscle tissue.

Balance and Coordination: Balance and coordination are important for sports along with sports activities sports, yoga, and each day practical actions. Assessing stability can contain reputation on one leg with eyes closed or appearing specific balance sports. Coordination may be evaluated through sports activities that require unique actions and manage, inclusive of throwing and catching a ball or appearing agility drills.

Resting Heart Rate and Blood Pressure: Monitoring your resting coronary heart fee and blood pressure can provide perception into your cardiovascular health. A decrease resting coronary heart charge is typically an illustration of better cardiovascular fitness, at the same time as immoderate blood strain may be a sign of underlying health problems. Regularly tracking the ones measurements will will let you discover any modifications or capacity problems.

It is essential to method health assessments with honesty, as they offer an correct mirrored picture of your modern-day-day health degree. By figuring out areas of energy and regions that need improvement, you may tailor your exercise ordinary to deal with precise goals and requirements. Additionally, health assessments feature a benchmark, allowing you to music improvement and make important changes in your schooling application through the years.

Choosing the proper sporting sports for muscle growth

Choosing the right physical video video games for muscle boom is an critical detail of designing an powerful exercising habitual. Whether youre a novice or an skilled lifter, expertise the thoughts at the back of exercising desire permit you to maximise your muscle profits and collect your health goals.

Compound vs. Isolation Exercises:

Compound wearing events contain multiple muscle corporations and joints, recruiting a larger fashion of muscle fibres and stimulating greater growth. Examples of compound carrying sports embody squats, deadlifts, bench press, and pull-ups. These sporting events are crucial for normal muscle development and must form the inspiration of your exercising ordinary. Isolation wearing activities, alternatively, purpose unique muscle tissues and joints and may be used to similarly decorate muscle development or cope with imbalances. Examples of isolation wearing sports consist of bicep curls, tricep extensions, and leg extensions. While isolation bodily activities have their region, prioritise compound actions to maximise muscle growth.

Exercise Variations:

Within every exercising elegance (compound or isolation), there are various exercise versions to select from. For example, squats can be completed with a barbell, dumbbells, or the use of a leg press device. Each variation gives a barely one in every of a kind stimulus to the muscle mass, difficult them from distinct angles and intensities. Incorporating numerous exercising variations into your normal allows save you plateaus, keeps your sporting events exciting, and promotes balanced muscle improvement.

Progressive Overload:

Progressive overload is the precept of little by little growing the pressure located at the muscle agencies over time to promote muscle boom. To benefit this, you want to pick out sports that allow you to regularly boom the burden or resistance youre the usage of. Free weight bodily sports like barbell squats or dumbbell bench press are excellent alternatives for current overload considering that you can effects alter the load. Machines, cables, and resistance bands also can be powerful, but they will have boundaries in terms of converting the resistance. Incorporate sporting activities into your normal that provide room for contemporary overload to stimulate muscle increase usually.

Balance and Symmetry:

Achieving balanced muscle improvement and symmetry is vital for each aesthetics and beneficial strength. When deciding on carrying occasions, remember the muscle tissue youre targeting and make sure youre incorporating actions that work all muscle corporations calmly. Neglecting wonderful muscle agencies can result in imbalances, that could boom the risk of harm and keep away from commonplace improvement. For instance, if you recognition absolutely on chest sports activities and forget approximately your back, it can result in rounded shoulders and horrific posture. Aim for a well-rounded routine that goals all essential muscle organizations.

Individual Needs and Goals:

Every person has particular goals and dreams almost approximately muscle growth. Factors together with schooling experience, fitness degree, body type, and personal selections have to be taken under consideration at the same time as choosing physical sports activities. For novices, its vital to cognizance on learning the essential compound physical video games and regularly improvement from there. Intermediate and superior lifters can encompass greater superior strategies, which includes supersets, drop devices, or plyometric physical activities, to mission their muscles in addition. If you have got were given particular weaknesses or areas you want to beautify, you may tailor your exercising choice for this reason.

Injury History and Limitations:

Consider any previous injuries or limitations you could have whilst selecting bodily games. Some bodily video games can also exacerbate present injuries or positioned undue pressure on advantageous joints. Its crucial to be aware of your frame and artwork with a qualified professional, which incorporates a bodily therapist or personal instructor, to decide which sports activities activities are regular and suitable for you. They assist you to alter bodily games or suggest alternatives in an effort to will let you art work spherical your limitations even as despite the fact that selling muscle increase.

Workout Variety and Progression:

To hold making development and stimulating muscle growth, its critical to vary your exercise routines and always undertaking your muscle mass. Incorporate one-of-a-kind sporting sports, rep ranges, and schooling strategies into your habitual to preserve your muscle groups guessing. Gradually growth the intensity or quantity of your exercising workout routines over time to provide a revolutionary stimulus. By incorporating variety and development, you may avoid plateaus and ensure ongoing muscle increase.

Structuring your exercise physical activities for most perfect outcomes

Structuring your exercises for greatest consequences is a important detail of any health recurring. Whether your cause is to gather muscle, decorate cardiovascular staying energy, shed kilos, or beautify normal health, an powerful exercise shape assist you to maximise your efforts and achieve your desired effects.

Chapter 15: Progressive Overload and Training Intensity

Understanding the precept of revolutionary overload

Understanding the principle of contemporary-day overload is essential for everyone trying to maximise their health profits and gain excellent outcomes from their training software program application. Progressive overload is a critical precept in exercising technological knowledge that bureaucracy the basis for power and muscle improvement. By often growing the wishes positioned on the body, individuals can continuously challenge their muscle mass and stimulate boom over time.

The principle of modern overload may be summarised as follows: To make enhancements in electricity, patience, or muscle period, an individual ought to usually boom the desires located on their frame via severa manner, which include developing resistance, extent, frequency, or depth in their sporting events. This precept applies to all forms of exercise, collectively with weightlifting, cardiovascular education, or maybe flexibility sporting occasions.

The human frame is relatively adaptable and green at appearing the duties it is often exposed to. When you first start an exercise application, your body research massive enhancements in power and commonplace ordinary performance due to the ultra-modern stimulus it encounters. However, over time, the frame turns into conversant within the desires positioned on it, and the preliminary earnings begin to plateau. This is wherein the precept of revolutionary overload turns into crucial.

Progressive overload can be finished thru numerous techniques, each of which goals a super element of education. Lets discover some of the most commonplace strategies used to use cutting-edge overload:

Increasing resistance: This approach includes which includes extra weight to your physical games. For example, in electricity training, frequently developing the quantity of weight lifted in the course of physical activities like squats, bench presses, or bicep curls will stress your muscle companies to adapt and grow more potent.

Increasing quantity: Volume refers to the overall quantity of hard work performed in a training session, typically measured thru using the widespread style of gadgets and repetitions completed. By growing the quantity, you could offer a extra stimulus for muscle growth. This may be achieved via together with extra gadgets, reps, or sports activities for your regular.

Increasing frequency: Frequency refers to how often you carry out a particular exercise or training session. Increasing the frequency allows for more not unusual stimulation of the muscles, enhancing their boom and model. However, its vital to stability frequency with ok rest and recuperation to prevent overtraining.

Increasing intensity: Intensity refers to the level of strive or problem of an workout. It can be manipulated via changing variables together with the fee of motion, decreasing rest periods, or incorporating advanced schooling techniques like drop devices or supersets. Increasing intensity worrying conditions the muscle mass in new techniques, fundamental to more variations.

Manipulating workout variables: Apart from resistance, quantity, frequency, and intensity, distinct exercising variables may be modified to introduce modern overload. These encompass changing the sort of movement, changing the pace of the movement, the usage of particular exercise variations, or enforcing superior education techniques like pyramids or negatives.

Its critical to be aware that the software program of cutting-edge overload want to be sluggish and systematic. Rapidly developing the intensity or quantity without taking into consideration suitable enough version and recovery can bring about overuse injuries, burnout, or a plateau in development. Progression should be individualised, thinking about elements collectively with fitness degree, training experience, and personal desires.

Additionally, modern-day overload isn't confined to just electricity training. It can be applied to important sorts of exercising, which consist of cardiovascular training. For instance, gradually growing the space, length, or depth of your aerobic exercise workout routines will always project your cardiovascular device, major to superior staying power and health.

Manipulating schooling intensity for muscle hypertrophy

Muscle hypertrophy, usually referred to as muscle growth, is a way that takes location in response to education stimuli and is encouraged via various factors, which includes training depth. Manipulating education depth is a crucial detail of designing an effective muscle hypertrophy utility.

Importance of Training Intensity for Muscle Hypertrophy:

Training intensity is a degree of the try exerted in the course of resistance schooling. It refers back to the relative load or percentage of an humans one-repetition maximum (1RM) that is lifted in some unspecified time in the future of a given workout. Training intensity plays a big position in promoting muscle hypertrophy because of the subsequent motives:

a. Mechanical Tension: Mechanical anxiety, or the stress completed to the muscles for the duration of resistance schooling, is a primary stimulus for muscle increase. Higher schooling intensities normally result in more mechanical tension, which activates molecular pathways worried in muscle protein synthesis and mobile permutations.

b. Motor Unit Recruitment: Motor gadgets are corporations of muscle fibres and the motor neuron that controls them. Higher training intensities recruit a wider variety of motor gadgets, leading to more muscle fibres being activated. This recruitment of a bigger muscle tissues contributes to hypertrophy.

c. Metabolic Stress: Resistance education at better intensities can motive metabolic stress, characterized by way of the usage of using the buildup of metabolites, such as lactate and hydrogen ions, within the muscle. This metabolic strain has been associated with hypertrophic variations, together with an increase in anabolic hormone launch and muscle fibre swelling.

Methods to Manipulate Training Intensity:

To optimise muscle hypertrophy, it is crucial to control training intensity strategically. Here are a few strategies typically employed:

a. Percentage of 1RM: This approach entails prescribing sporting sports and hundreds based on a percentage of an human beings 1RM. Higher opportunities (70-eighty 5% of 1RM) are typically used for hypertrophy-focused education, while lower opportunities are greater suitable for electricity or endurance schooling. Adjusting the percentage of 1RM allows for revolutionary overload, wherein the intensity is step by step accelerated over the years to stimulate persisted muscle growth.

b. Repetition Range: Another manner to govern education depth is thru the use of a selected repetition variety. Moderate to excessive repetition ranges (e.G., 6-12 repetitions steady with set) are normally used for hypertrophy schooling, as they bring about every mechanical tension and metabolic strain. Lower repetition stages (e.G., 1-5 repetitions in keeping with set) are frequently utilised for energy-focused education, whilst higher tiers (e.G., 12-20 repetitions in keeping with set) can aim muscular staying energy.

c. Tempo: Manipulating the tempo, or pace of motion, can have an effect on education intensity. Different tempo prescriptions, which encompass slow eccentric (lowering) or explosive concentric (lifting) levels, can regulate the time below anxiety and growth the problem of an exercise. Slower tempos generally growth the time muscle mass spend below anxiety, potentially improving hypertrophic responses.

d. Training Techniques: Various schooling strategies can be hired to manipulate training depth. For example, drop units include appearing a set to failure, then without delay lowering the burden and continuing for brought repetitions. Supersets involve acting wearing sports lower again-to-decrease returned with minimal rest. These techniques growth training density and metabolic stress, maximum vital to stronger hypertrophy responses.

Considerations for Maximising Muscle Hypertrophy:

While manipulating training depth is vital for muscle hypertrophy, it is vital to hold in thoughts the following factors for maximum suitable effects:

a. Individual Differences: Training intensity need to be tailor-made to an human beings fitness level, enjoy, and goals. Novices might also gain from starting with decrease intensities to expand proper shape and technique in advance than progressing to higher intensities.

b. Progressive Overload: To sell ongoing muscle growth, schooling intensity ought to be regularly extended over the years. Gradually consisting of load, repetitions, or trouble guarantees that the muscular tissues maintain to conform and increase.

c. Periodization: Incorporating periodization into your training plan is important for prolonged-term improvement. This consists of dividing training into particular ranges, collectively with hypertrophy, electricity, and deloading levels. Manipulating schooling intensity inner every segment and transitioning amongst them optimises muscle hypertrophy and prevents plateauing.

d. Recovery and Nutrition: Adequate rest and recovery are critical for muscle growth. Intense schooling locations strain on the muscle tissue, and they need time to repair and adapt. Additionally, proper vitamins, which include enough protein consumption, plays a crucial function in assisting muscle hypertrophy.

Chapter 16: The Perfect Repetition and Technique

Proper form and method for each workout

Proper form and approach are critical in terms of acting sports. Whether youre a novice or an skilled athlete, the usage of correct form no longer quality maximises the effectiveness of the exercising but additionally enables save you accidents.

Squats:

Stand collectively together with your toes shoulder-width aside, ft slightly grew to become out.

Keep your chest up, shoulders decrease again, and engage your middle.

Initiate the motion thru pushing your hips again and bending your knees.

Lower your body as although youre sitting once more proper proper into a chair, making sure your knees live in keeping with your toes.

Descend until your thighs are parallel to the ground or barely beneath.

Drive via your heels and push your hips beforehand to go returned to the beginning role.

Deadlifts:

Stand together with your toes hip-width apart, ft pointing in advance, and the barbell over your midfoot.

Bend down and grip the barbell with an overhand or blended grip (one hand overhand, one underhand).

Keep your decrease lower back proper now, chest up, and have interaction your middle.

Drive thru your heels, push the ground away, and lift the bar with the aid of extending your hips and knees.

As you convey, preserve the barbell close to your body, and maintain a unbiased spine.

Stand up tall, certainly extending your hips and knees, and squeeze your glutes on the top.

Lower the bar via reversing the motion, preserving your decrease returned right away sooner or later of.

Bench Press:

Lie flat on a bench collectively along side your toes firmly planted at the ground.

Position your hands slightly wider than shoulder-width aside on the barbell.

Lift the bar off the rack, lock your elbows, and maintain it straight away above your chest.

Lower the bar in a managed way on your mid-chest, keeping your elbows at a 45-diploma attitude in your body.

Pause in short, then push the bar again up, completely extending your arms with out locking your elbows.

Keep your feet grounded, preserve a mild arch to your lower all over again, and engage your middle at some point of the exercise.

Overhead Press:

Stand along side your feet shoulder-width apart, center engaged, and maintain a barbell or dumbbells at shoulder stage.

Press the load overhead with the aid of extending your fingers and truly extending your elbows.

As you raise, preserve your core tight, and avoid arching your lower back excessively.

Lower the weight all over again to the start characteristic with manage, ensuring it doesnt touch your body.

Throughout the workout, maintain a right away posture and keep away from leaning backward.

Lunges:

Stand at the side of your feet hip-width aside.

Take a step forward together together with your right foot, bending each knees to create a 90-degree thoughts-set.

Keep your all over again right away, chest up, and interact your middle.

Push through your right heel to return to the begin feature.

Repeat with the left leg, alternating elements with every rep.

Maintain manipulate within the route of the motion, fending off excessive ahead knee movement and preserving your torso upright.

Understanding the significance of complete form of movement

Full variety of motion (ROM) refers back to the whole movement ability of a joint or a collection of joints inside the body. It encompasses the capability to move a frame detail thru its whole range with out guidelines or boundaries. Whether its a easy motion like bending your elbow or a complex workout like a deep squat, having a whole shape of motion is vital for maximum best bodily feature and normal fitness.

Here are numerous motives why know-how and prioritising entire kind of motion is critical:

Injury Prevention: Maintaining a full sort of movement lets in lessen the chance of injuries. When a joint has constrained mobility, compensations also can additionally occur, putting excessive stress on surrounding muscle mass, tendons, and ligaments. Over time, this may purpose imbalances, muscle strains, joint instability, and extended susceptibility to injuries. By regularly strolling for your ROM, you could beautify joint stability, decorate muscle coordination, and reduce the possibility of injuries.

Enhanced Performance: Full kind of motion is critical for most beneficial athletic general general overall performance. Many sports activities sports and sports require a sizable kind of movements, which incorporates engaging in, twisting, leaping, and bending. Having accurate flexibility and mobility in the joints lets in athletes to transport more correctly, generate greater power, and carry out complex movements with precision. Whether youre a professional athlete or someone who enjoys enjoyment activities, enhancing your ROM can enhance your not unusual traditional universal performance and amusement of physical sports.

Functional Movement: Full form of movement is carefully tied to functional motion, which refers to the capability to perform normal obligations and not using a hassle and overall performance. Simple movements like bending proper all the way down to tie your shoes, accomplishing overhead to seize an item from a shelf, or getting up from a chair require a whole style of motion in multiple joints. Without desirable sufficient ROM, those number one moves can grow to be hard and uncomfortable. By keeping and enhancing your flexibility, you could make certain that you could perform each day responsibilities with out useless obstacles or soreness.

Muscle Balance and Symmetry: Full type of movement plays a crucial characteristic in accomplishing muscle balance and symmetry. When powerful muscle businesses are tight or shortened, they may pull on opposing muscular tissues, causing imbalances. These imbalances can lead to postural problems, joint misalignment, and chronic pain.

Chapter 17: Training Frequency and Recovery

Determining the maximum ideal education frequency for muscle increase

Determining the gold general education frequency for muscle increase is a topic of excellent hobby and debate inside the health and bodybuilding companies. While there may be no person-length-suits-all solution, severa elements need to be considered at the same time as designing an powerful training software, consisting of person desires, training experience, recovery capacity, and popular life-style. In this chat, we're capable of discover diverse elements of schooling frequency and its effect on muscle increase.

Before delving into the statistics, its vital to understand the concept of revolutionary overload. Progressive overload refers to grade by grade growing the needs placed at the muscle groups to stimulate boom and model. By constantly difficult the muscular tissues through resistance training, they're pressured to adapt via becoming more potent and large over time.

Training frequency refers to how often you educate a particular muscle or muscle organisation internal a given time frame, usually measured in classes in keeping with week. The frequency can vary from individual to individual, and locating the most education frequency includes finding the proper stability amongst education stimulus and recovery.

Here are severa key factors to consider while figuring out the first-rate schooling frequency for muscle boom:

Training Experience: Beginners usually have the capability to get better quicker and can advantage from a better schooling frequency, as their muscle tissues aren't acquainted with excessive wearing occasions. A frequency of two-3 times constant with week for each muscle organization can be effective within the initial tiers.

Advanced Lifters: As people development of their schooling, their healing potential can also moreover moreover lower, requiring longer periods of relaxation. Advanced lifters regularly advantage from reducing schooling frequency to permit for extra immoderate durations and advanced healing time. Training every muscle institution 1-2 times in step with week might be more appropriate for knowledgeable lifters.

Volume and Intensity: The extent and intensity of your workouts play a great feature in figuring out schooling frequency. If you carry out excessive-amount workout routines with some of gadgets and sports activities activities, it is able to be essential to permit for additonal healing time between training. Conversely, if your sporting activities are decrease in amount and intensity, you will be able to teach extra regularly.

www.ingramcontent.com/pod-product-compliance
Lightning Source LLC
Chambersburg PA
CBHW071444080526
44587CB00014B/1988